A CANADIAN WOMAN'S WAY

LIVING SLIM

LILLIAN SALMON

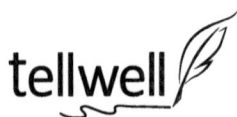

Tellwell Talent

www.tellwell.ca

ISBN

978-0-2288-1046-9 (Hardcover)

978-0-2288-1045-2 (Paperback)

978-0-2288-1044-5 (eBook)

DEDICATION

"In my mother's house, there were always apples."

This book is dedicated to my mother Edna Jean (White) Scott.

A tiny, slim, intelligent person, she was the most important influence on my life. I hope she knew how much I valued all she taught me about life.

TABLE OF CONTENTS

CHAPTER 1

Let's Take a Walk

Walk into any mainstream Canadian supermarket and you will see shelves of fruits and tabletops of vegetables.

Row after row of onion, squash, potato and tomato. Mound after mound of lemon, pineapple, melon and grape. Overflowing cases of leafy greens, herbs, and celery stalks.

But now, look for the apples.

Suddenly, it's not a bin, a bag, a box or a row. Suddenly, you see row after row, stacked displays, piles of bags, overflowing bushel baskets, an entire long display case with more at the end. Ten times, twenty times the space dedicated to the avocado, the kiwi, or the banana.

And that's the first of many reasons Canadian women can manage to live slim. No one puts on weight – ever – eating and enjoying the apple. And in Canada, we do enjoy lots of them.

Sadly, however, our Canadian world is also crammed full of simply awful food and epidemic over-eating. And for every slim Canadian woman packing an apple for lunch, there is another packing on more pounds than she would like.

Canada doesn't stand alone in this regard. The World Health Organization noted, in 2018, that obesity worldwide has nearly tripled since 1975.[1] *Tripled!*

And Canada's Public Health Agency now says fully 64% of Canadians over the age of eighteen are either overweight or obese.[2]

Fortunately, it doesn't *have* to be this way.

And, sure, while we can consider the habits of women in France, the Mediterranean, Asia, or anywhere else in our efforts to live slim, Canadian women also have our very own collection of habits and beliefs – some new, many old – that can keep us as slim and as healthy as we wish to be for our entire lives.

This book celebrates this.

It also explores those sometimes unrecognized habits and beliefs, starting with the ones I learned in my slim Canadian mother's home in Nova Scotia's fertile Annapolis Valley – where there were always apples.

Make no mistake, however. This book is not an effort in praise of model-thinness. Look elsewhere if that is what you seek. This book is about becoming, and remaining, as slim and trim as you want to be. As slim and trim as is good for you. And as slim and trim as suits your build.

Women everywhere always know at just what weight we feel best. We also know when that extra five, 12, or 35 pounds, resting uncomfortably somewhere on our body, is just the amount we don't want to have. I've been there – twice – and I remember.

Understand, as well, that for some women more specialized medical help may be needed.

Appetite and metabolism, like every other bodily function, can become disordered to the point of illness and can then require a different kind of help. If that is the case for you, by all means read this book, take from it what you will – especially, my hope would be that you take encouragement – but if you need more help, do seek it out. Don't give up!

So, exactly what were the habits and beliefs that allowed my mother to live slim for a lifetime – seemingly without trying? What are the secrets that keep many other Canadian women trim and healthy as well?

The apple is as good a place as any to start.

CHAPTER 2

The Apple...and all of that

It was a crisp fall day when I carried one of my first heavy loads of groceries-for-one to my tiny room-for-one through the leafy, tree-lined streets of London, Ontario. I was in my early twenties and just getting used to living on my own in that university town about 120 miles west of Toronto.

I had selected fully enough – and more than enough – to carry that day.

But, as I finished up my shopping in that London supermarket, I couldn't resist adding to my cart that four-pound bag of luscious looking apples. They were so glowing in their autumn freshness. They promised so much juicy delight. They spoke to me so deeply of faraway home and family.

I lived to regret it all that heavy, arm-aching walk home.

How many times I had to set my load down on the sidewalk. How many times I said to myself: never again. How many times I wondered if I would actually make it. And all the way home I knew it was that bag of apples that had tipped the scales into more than I could manage.

But it was a bag of apples that, against all common sense, I couldn't resist.

I'm sure a large part of the reason I still carry that memory is because of the pain that drilled itself into my arms that day.

But what I also remember is the wonderful, emotional allure of those apples: their promise of satisfaction; the sense of rightness of having a bag of apples in my solitary room, so far from home.

For in my mother's house, there were always apples.

A great deal of them came from the family farm on my father's side of the family. At that time, the farm contained an old but still-producing orchard, bordered by country roads, at the eastern edge of the Annapolis Valley. Many also came from roadside farmers' markets in that same fertile valley where we lived.

But as seasonal offerings passed, many came, as they do for most of us now, from our nearest grocery store.

Winter, summer, spring or fall, Canadians can count on apples. Thank goodness for modern cold storage. In my father's time, the apples were kept in the farm's below-ground cold cellar, along with turnips, carrots, and potatoes. Yes, they did last until spring that way, but barely.

In our time, however, better storage methods – and, of course, imports – mean we have good-tasting apples year round. And the disproportionate amount of real estate devoted to apples, in every Canadian grocery store from Sackville to Saskatoon, attests to their popularity.

Nova Scotia's lush Annapolis Valley certainly was – and remains – quite a bit more focused on apples than the rest of the country.

Not content with merely cultivating apples, residents of this verdant agricultural region have long cultivated an apple culture that includes an Apple Blossom Festival each spring with Apple Blossom princesses, parades, floats, and many related celebrations.

Few sights can top the loveliness of the valley's delicate, frothy, flowering apple orchards every spring. Personally, I have completely mixed feelings as I see some of those gorgeous, hilly orchards metamorphose, in recent times, into the stretching, sinuous lines of flourishing vineyards.

Growing up in Wolfville, a small university town in the valley, I absorbed this apple culture. I became fixed with the idea that biting into a crisp, beautiful apple was a perfect delight; that a bowl of glossy apples was a visual treat; that the humble Russet apple – humble only in appearance – was a triumph of taste and pleasure.

We did indeed hear the old saying: "An apple a day keeps the doctor away." And we were indeed encouraged to think of the apple as the ultimate snack.

I took for granted my mother's stewed apples, baked in the oven, skins on, and served simply with a drizzle of cream. I also took for granted her homemade or store-bought applesauce for dessert and as a garnish for salty, crackling roast pork. And my young life saw me enjoy many a delicious homemade apple pie or apple crisp.

Then there was the apple creation I didn't have at home; the creation I sampled deep in the dark of the New Brunswick woods one late summer's night.

I was not yet twenty, driving homeward with friends, to Nova Scotia from a summer job in Quebec. Our route was following the great national reach of the Trans-Canada Highway.

My friends had planned a one-night stopover to visit an older friend, a former teacher, now retired and happily immersed in country life.

I still remember all three of us watching for signs to make the correct turn-off in the lowering darkness, checking to see if we could find our way to a country road we did not know.

Was it this road? Was it that one? Did we have the right directions really? Had we missed a turn? Wooded New Brunswick roads can all look very, very much alike to novice travellers once the sun sets. We didn't have a Plan B.

It was almost dark by the time we found the correct turn-off, quite dark when we found the correct secondary road, and fully dark when we found the correct driveway. But there, in the darkness, was the house, glowing with lights and welcome.

As we stepped inside, the complex aromas of a traditional, roasted ham dinner greeted our weary senses. There was the large dining table beautifully set with a white tablecloth and gleaming silver. Dinner was ready and waiting. We were waiting and ready for it!

Few experiences have so perfectly mixed relief, tiredness, appreciation, and hunger as they were melded for me that night, sealing my memories of that warm home in the New Brunswick woods. Sealing, as well, the memory of my first-ever taste of homemade crabapple preserves.

Glowing deep pink, sweet and tart, studded with cloves, outstanding in taste and appearance, they were served, with pride, as a garnish for the ham. Later we saw them, beautiful in their jars, along with our host's other homemade preserves, lining her orderly pantry shelves.

I've mentioned that our host was a retired teacher, but I've not mentioned her area of teaching expertise.

She taught what we used to call Home Economics, a dry and unimaginative label indeed, that doesn't come close to capturing the satisfyingly wonderful management of the household arts, especially in all things related to food, of which she was a skilled and devoted practitioner.

Her meticulously crafted crabapple preserves were an apple delight my mother didn't serve, one I wasn't used to, but one that stands in my mind as exquisite perfection.

That night we enjoyed a slow food meal with all the slow food trimmings – long before such a concept was needed, considered, or dreamt of.

A few years later, when I began to enjoy the food columns of a certain Madame Jehane Benoît, Canada and Quebec's *grande dame* of cuisine, it was often that homestead, in the New Brunswick woods, that correspondingly and simultaneously came to mind.

In Nova Scotia today, as the annual apple season commences, early Gravensteins are snapped up quickly by women in the know for winter applesauce. Friends actually make a point of telling each other when they're in the stores!

And in Ontario, where I live, surely nothing beats the sharp, sweet tang of the "early Macs" which appear in our supermarkets, and then disappear far too quickly. I still watch for the short selling interval of the increasingly rare Russet apple, which has been crowded out by so many new varieties.

Autumn "pick-your-own" apple gatherings, in orchards from the Niagara region to British Columbia's Okanagan, are popular, Canadian, family events.

In Quebec, locally brewed apple cider provides a crisp and sparkling counterpoint to many a well-turned crepe.

In my mother's house, there were always apples.

But there was something far more important that accompanied those apples as well. And that's the "all of that" situation referenced in the title of this chapter.

In my mother's house, what accompanied those apples was the belief that fresh food is good food, that real tastes are the best tastes, and that gifts of the earth are to be cherished, savoured, and treated with care.

Foremost among those gifts of the earth: fresh fruits and vegetables. *Not* chips, or pop, or any other dreadful variation of junk food.

Turning this belief into habits of living continues to be the first and most important practice that allows Canadian women to live slim. It's the first and most important idea underpinning any effort to be trim and healthy. And it's the first and most important acknowledgement required in any attempt to stem the obesity epidemic worldwide.

It is simply extremely difficult to put on weight when we're eating plenty of high-quality fresh fruits and vegetables, and when our minds and taste buds are trained to fully embrace their natural and satisfying flavours.

By the same token, it is generally easy to stay slim and healthy when these items stay at the top of the list of foods we value.

This was the first essential belief and habit I learned at my mother's table. And this belief and habit is at the core of most patterns of healthy food consumption in Canada past and present.

My mother was born in 1911 and grew up in the small, port city of St. John's, Newfoundland. She met my dad while he was serving there, as a Navy chaplain, during the Second World War. Sturdily handsome, this farm boy turned United Church minister quickly swept my mother off her schoolteacher feet – in the nicest possible way.

"So," wrote his longtime friend and college mate, in decidedly unministerial language, "I hear the Nova Scotian wolf has captured the Newfoundland prize. Congratulations."

Their wedding portrait shows their low-key wartime wedding. Both of them beaming. He, in his formal Navy gear and clerical collar. She, in her trim and beautifully tailored suit, with her bouquet of flowers.

Their happy marriage was soon enlivened by the arrival of my sister, my brother, and me.

My mum was the product of several migratory waves of individuals who arrived in this land, mostly from southwest England, in the 18th and 19th century. Her forebears set up businesses, built ships, became sea captains, raised families, and contributed to politics, community and social life.

Hard-working and pragmatic, like most immigrants who hope to make a good life in a new place, they also attempted to preserve the best of the traditions they did not want to leave behind. One of those traditions was this practical and almost respectful attitude toward real food.

Always, my mother ensured we had fruits of various types in our household. Always, we had vegetables. Rarely, did we ever have chips or pop, or junk food of any kind.

And believe me, my mother's grocery shopping choices, in a small Atlantic Canadian town during the 1950s and '60s of my youth, were vastly more limited than the options available to Canadian women today.

Broccoli, to take one example, was virtually unknown when I was young. Head lettuce was the order of the day: tired, tasteless, and boring. Spinach, for some reason, always tasted awful. Now that I think of it, perhaps it was tinned. I knew nothing of zucchinis, eggplants, or peppers. Mushrooms were of the tinned variety only.

But we did have other choices: wonderful foods we simply

took for granted. Foods that are still widely, cheaply, and readily available across Canada in our grocery stores, and some that are downright trendy in Canadian restaurants today.

Take fresh beets. A mainstay of our lives growing up. But certainly not found on many restaurant menus 45 years ago when I first ventured into the then-rather-limited, Canadian, dining-out scene.

At home, we often had them simply steamed, served with bit of salt, and sometimes a skimming of butter. Some family members found them incomplete without a splash of vinegar. Sweet, silky and delicious, beets remain one of my favourite vegetables.

It was also completely routine for us to have them pickled, sometimes spiked with cloves, providing a delightful bit of summer to brighten many a winter meal.

Today, a person can sit in the heart of downtown Ottawa, on a brilliant spring day with the Peace Tower in view, Parliament a few steps away, streets and sidewalks filled with bustling lunch crowds, tulips blooming, and the sun shining, and, in the middle of all this, a person can enjoy a delicious beet salad *alfresco*. Served in a busy, street-side cafe, it is nestled on arugula, circled with cranberries, sprinkled generously with fresh walnuts, topped with gorgeous goat cheese from Quebec, and lightly dressed with oil and lemon. Every mouthful of that beet salad goes down well. And not a mouthful of that salad would sideline the efforts of any Canadian woman endeavouring to live slim.

This type of meal was unheard of in Canada 45 years ago. But this is the sort of fabulous food Canadian women now take for granted in many a small restaurant right across the country. This is also the sort of fabulous food Canadian women can put together at home with relative ease. And this is the sort of fabulous food anyone can now find in and around that same small Atlantic

Canadian town where my mother shopped.

Now, consider the cabbage. Surely, one of the most ordinary and common vegetables found in any Canadian supermarket whether in my mother's time or now. It's available year round, is pretty well always of good quality, and now usually shares shelf space with the delicate Savoy, the red/purple, or the Chinese varieties.

Millions of Canadian women besides me must surely enjoy cabbage. Because these round, heavy clunkers are constantly being replenished on the produce shelves.

Cabbage is an absolute mainstay for soup. All of the varieties are great, all year round, for stir-fries. It's perfect steamed to wilted sweetness and served plain with a skim of butter or oil. And, of course, it's essential for coleslaw whether you enjoy coleslaw à la mayonnaise or à la vinaigrette.

No Canadian woman puts on pounds eating cabbage. Imagine, just imagine, how very much cabbage you would have to eat to do that!

Sometimes, of a Saturday, my mother used to cook so-called Jiggs' Dinner. A souvenir of her Newfoundland upbringing, Jiggs' Dinner is cured, salted beef, slow-stewed (she used a pressure cooker) with lots of cabbage chunks, carrots, onions, turnips, and large pieces of potatoes.

We loved it. And that salty, soft, and admittedly vastly over-cooked texture is still one of my fondest associations for cooked cabbage. Some southern American cooking traditions have a similar habit with green beans: a long, slow, salty overcook that, if you like it, you really like it.

But I'm a product of my time, and my adult life doesn't include quite the same degree of cured meats as my mother's.

So my normal cabbage cook-ups involve very thinly sliced

cabbage – green, purple, or Savoy, it doesn't matter – steamed to doneness with a splatter of oil, a very small splash of water, a shake of salt, and a sprinkle of sugar. I use as little water as possible when cooking any vegetable, the better to retain its flavour. Wilted, tender, sweet, and delicious, cabbage cooked like this in my house often gets a sprinkle of caraway seeds scattered into the mix as well.

I remember my first few months in Toronto, in the late sixties, when my youthful palate first discovered the falafel sandwich. It was cranked out with incredibly efficient dispatch – and a certain amount of theatrical flair – from a busy, basic and noisy storefront on Spadina Avenue.

I'd never tasted such a combination before. Those interesting little balls of ground-up chickpeas slathered with what I still remember as the best and most generous dollop of sliced and seasoned cabbage I had ever tasted. All bound up in a thin and flexible flatbread that certainly did not come from the Annapolis Valley.

"What is this?" my taste buds murmured. And I went back for more.

Beets, cabbage, turnip, parsnip, onions, squash, carrots, and potatoes formed the backbone of our vegetable offerings during the winter months of my Nova Scotian upbringing. Their warm, sweet, familiar aromas, usually enhanced by being roasted in the oven alongside beef, pork, or chicken, greeted us regularly as we kids stomped back into the house late in the afternoon, snow falling off our boots, cheeks and hands cold from the outdoors, and appetites ready for our winter meals.

Just to linger with parsnips for a moment, theirs was a flavour I couldn't accept as a child. Not quite like a carrot, not quite like a turnip, I couldn't see their value. But, as an adult, I certainly do. And it's a delight to see them making a comeback on the Canadian restaurant scene.

I recently discovered a tiny, perfect serving of delicate cream of parsnip soup, presented in the middle of a sampling platter, in a modest but wonderful restaurant along Toronto's Danforth strip. It was outstanding. In many Canadian restaurants it has become not at all uncommon to discover parsnips served among scrumptious sides of roasted root vegetables.

The winters of my youth may have been limited in terms of vegetable offerings, but in the summer we enjoyed fresh and flavourful lettuce from farmers' markets, from our own backyard, and from our family's farm. We knew the taste of homegrown parsley, tender beet greens, silky Swiss chard and shock-your-mouth, nippy radishes, fresh from the earth.

Nowadays, the variety of fresh produce and good food available to Canadian women just about anywhere in the country is just about fantastic: bok choy; avocados; celeriac; sweet potatoes; assorted yams; an amazing array of fresh leafy greens, including the tender sorts and also kale, Swiss chard and beet greens; multiple types of mushrooms; zucchini; fresh parsley and a blizzard of fresh herbs all year round. Cherry tomatoes are a personal favourite, retaining, to my taste, the essentials of the true and delightful tomato flavour better than the larger ones. Interesting olives are everywhere. Ditto for delicious fresh nuts.

The list just keeps growing, pushed by mushrooming availability and the expectations of a population keen to enjoy all the fresh flavours of the world.

As for fruit, don't get me started: as a child, I never tasted fresh pineapple. But local, seasonal fruits were, of course, fabulous. Apples, naturally. But also blueberries – best enjoyed when just gathered and still warm from the hot August sun. Those I got to savour, hand-picked, at the family farm. It was hard for me to fill my picking containers, I ate so many.

Today, Nova Scotia's Annapolis Valley remains one of the most delightful places on earth to pick your own blueberries. I am still so in love with these small fruits that, here in Ontario, I buy box after box, all summer long. Even as I could barely resist that bag of apples years ago, I can still barely resist a grocery store display of these plump, little blue treasures.

Back in the valley of my youth, we also had pears. Sweet and intoxicating for the short period they were at their best, they were enjoyed annually in massive amounts.

A recent visit to Nova Scotia's farming village of Grand Pré, the heartland of French Acadia and now protected as a UNESCO world heritage site, saw me waxing ecstatic over a delicious homemade pear and ginger conserve served at a small, local eatery. So much so that I found myself asking for a few extra servings to take home!

We also enjoyed strawberries, much sweeter and more intense in flavour than generally found now; silky, tantalizing peaches; and luscious raspberries, blackberries, gooseberries and plums. All of these treasures were only available in season. Many were home-preserved for enjoyment in the winter.

My mother did a limited amount of home canning. She also made pickles. And she certainly made jam. Strawberry was a favourite, as was her tart but delicious damson plum preserve.

My memory holds that image of her still: cheeks flushed from the heat and effort, the soft waves of her hair curled from the steam, her body small-framed and focused in her kitchen apron, and her large wooden spoon in hand, stirring that very large pot as the scented steam rose deliciously, telling us jam was in process.

Whatever didn't make it into the jam jars remained on a dish, warm and sweet, to be used up immediately. Her large wooden spoon remains in my possession to this day, decorating my kitchen wall.

Home-freezing was growing in popularity during that time. Many folks in my agriculture-rich region were investing in good-sized freezers to store their tender seasonal fruits and vegetables. Many a Canadian continues to do this, despite the increased availability of good, commercially frozen products.

One Ontario friend recently showed me her large stash of plastic baggies, filled with frozen, cut-up Ontario peaches that she had put by, as my aunt on the farm might have done, for her breakfasts during our cold Canadian winters when the quality of the imports simply cannot compete.

During the winter months of my youth, grocery stores stocked apples, oranges, grapefruit, bananas and grapes. Sometimes, pale-flavoured melons. And, oddly enough, quite a few whole coconuts, which we enjoyed immensely, learning to crack them with a hammer, drink the juice, and munch away on the soft, white flesh.

Nowadays, we all know the array of imported fruit that is available to us year round. Not all of it as complex and satisfying in taste as the varieties that don't have to travel great distances to reach us, but much of it very good anyway.

In my mother's house, our normal diet revolved around a solid array of fruits and vegetables every day. They were the unquestioned foundation of every meal. Fruit was always available for snacks, and also used in desserts. We never had any kind of sit-down dinner or lunch without vegetables making up a good half of our plate. Many of these items were simple to the point that we thought nothing of them. Some of them were of gourmet quality, but we didn't think of things that way.

And that is the way the engraining of habits takes place. In the case of good habits, it's a very good thing. In the case of bad habits, completely the reverse.

There was something deeply engrained in me that fall day, years ago, when I bought that 4-pound bag of apples, just for me alone.

Interestingly enough, although I have a very clear memory of that purchase – and the excruciating delivery – I have no memory at all of just how long it took me to get through that bagful.

But now the fundamental question: why, with so many Canadian food habits celebrating fruits and vegetables, and with such broad availability of these items today across our country, do some Canadian women carry more weight than they would like?

Why did I, with so many good, healthy eating habits engrained in me, did I nevertheless gain an uncomfortable 25-30 extra pounds in my late teens and early twenties?

Why, although each and every cultural group in our country can look to a relatively recent history of relatively healthy eating, do so many of us so easily forget those good and healthy habits and stray quite far from the kind of balanced diet that we know, deep down, we should be following?

In my opinion, one of the main reasons is that our normal eating patterns have been under attack, for many years now, by commercial food interests that make far more money from cheap and torturous combinations of salt, sugar, fat, and starch than from crunchy apples on a Sunday afternoon.

These dreadful combinations have been in our lives, for most of us, *our entire lives*, degrading our sense of taste, having us believe that hyped-up flavours are desirable over real ones, that empty calories can somehow compete with real nourishment, and that something sweet and coloured is better than water to quench our thirst. These items dupe us and leave us chronically hungry, without really knowing it, for the real thing.

This junk food – this *malbouffe* as Quebeckers would say – is marketed with a huge overlay of artificial emotion. It has to be, because there's not much else on which it can be marketed.

It reminds me of the counter-intuitive public relations advice I once heard: to sell the most questionable aspects of a political platform, a speechmaker need but raise his or her voice during that part of the speech. Speak more loudly. The questionable suddenly becomes certainty; the false becomes true.

We have been bombarded by loud and false voices in the marketing of junk food for generations. It now takes a conscious effort of will to deconstruct that bombardment, and to choose what is real, savoury, and delightful over a vast array of useless junk.

Despite the exceptionally good habits learned at my mother's table, I was not immune to the lure of fake food any more than any other Canadian woman growing up in my time.

Looking back, I believe it was the taste of sweet combined with fat that first led me astray. I adored the homemade desserts that were periodically available to me in my own home, and also in the homes of relatives. This quickly led on to purchased sweet items such as candy bars, commercially created bakery items, and varieties of ice cream. I won't name brand names, but I had my favourites in every area.

Looking back again, I think my attraction to salty and fatty items started a bit later. But again, I found myself quickly attracted and quickly consuming them to excess. I don't know how to say it more honestly. I edged toward readily available junk food. And junk food welcomed me with open arms. Despite the good, solid and healthy food environment in which I grew up.

Without question, commercial food interests have dominated our eating environment for a very long time. I have come to believe that the chemistry of our brains has been brutally overwhelmed by the kinds of food products we've been exposed to during this time. Whatever systems, signals or shortcuts our brain used for millennia to ensure our survival are now tricked and tricked again by wildly distorted flavours and easy energy fixes.

I believe this is what happened to me in my over-indulgence in certain food products that were not real foods, but rather artificially created concoctions that relied almost exclusively on sugar, fat, salt, and a lab full of chemicals to give them flavour.

Staying slim for me and for others in today's world is now very much a matter of re-tricking our brains, re-programming ourselves, and fighting fire with fire in order to appreciate real food.

Fortunately, for me, the lessons of my mother's house eventually resurfaced – with a bit of effort – and remained and grew throughout the rest of my life.

It wasn't particularly easy for me to lose the 25 pounds I needed to lose in my mid-twenties. But I worked at it, mainly with a low-calorie regime that cut out all desserts and junk foods. And I eventually succeeded.

But the truer, harder, more complete and far more important part was the lifelong choice I made to genuinely switch my focus to real foods, wonderful foods, foods of value as well as flavour.

This was the path I'd been shown as a child. This was my mother's path. This was truly *living* slim as opposed to dieting temporarily to become slim.

Despite some digressions, wobbles, hiccups and groans – notably another almost identical weight gain at midlife (more on that later) – this path, which values the true treasures of the earth as the true staples of one's diet became, for the most part, my own main true path as much as it was hers.

What I've discovered is that this has also been the case for many other slim Canadian women, however much we might sometimes stray. Many of us stay slim and healthy by cherishing the best of our respective cultural heritages while also broadening our scope to include the endless possibilities of wonderful, real food now available in Canada.

I still find myself munching on raw, cut carrots as I prepare dinner meals. Carrot sticks were a staple for my now-grown kids when they were young, and I continue to ensure there are carrot sticks ready when my young grandchildren arrive for a visit. I now also happily pay extra for the better-tasting, organically grown carrots available in my nearest supermarket.

I may be standing in my Toronto kitchen as I munch, but my mind routinely goes back to a wide-open and sun-drenched field, baking under a sweeping and still New Brunswick sky. A country road. The smell of grasses and earth. A distant reach of trees. A farm house at the end of a long driveway with a welcoming neighbour who had a peculiar and endlessly fascinating cuckoo clock.

All of that and more is recalled by the crisp, sweet taste of my citified carrot. Granted, not quite the indescribably nippy taste of the tiny carrots pulled from a kitchen garden just minutes before being munched by my seven-year-old self. But close enough.

Most of us have similar fruit and vegetable memories uniquely our own.

Consider the thin and delicate Asian-inspired soups of noodle, chicken, and vegetables, infused with the flavours of onion and garlic, which form an integral part of many a family meal at kitchen tables across our country.

Consider the Mediterranean-inspired pairing of Canadian green beans, pulled from an organic field or snapped from a tiny, sun-soaked, carefully-tended city garden, cooked up gently with fresh basil, olive oil, and tomato.

Consider the crates of mangoes shipped regularly from India, eagerly purchased at certain times of the year by Canadians whose affection for the fruit is as deeply held as mine for the apples of our homegrown September.

If, for whatever reason, we don't have such memories that celebrate the valuable complexity of fruits and vegetables, it is not — it is never — too late to create them. And it is likely essential to consciously do this if we have wandered too far into the unproductive habit of valuing fake food over the intrinsic pleasures of the real.

This concept seems simple but it's exceedingly strong: these gifts of authentic taste and treasure are the first and most important key to keeping us slim and healthy.

For some of us, this may mean sitting quietly and slowly enjoying the complex, sweet tang of a fresh peach or a bowl of raspberries as we unwind in the evening. It may mean sampling sliced baby zucchini — yellow or green — with some homemade yogurt dip when we think of a pick-me-up between meals. It may very happily mean creating main dishes with foods we especially enjoy such as eggplant, grilled peppers or delicious sweet potatoes. And it may also mean wowing our friends with the taste and texture of an amazing kale salad tossed with crunchy, toasted almonds and balsamic vinaigrette.

Certainly it does mean acknowledging — deeply and profoundly — that these items are more enjoyable, more delightful and more sparkling in taste than any junk food we could ever consume.

When we choose to celebrate and savour these delicate and varied flavours, when we focus our anticipatory thoughts of food, our celebrations and our quiet, personal enjoyments around them, we have very little problem with our weight.

We need to do this while we're losing weight. We need to do this while we're maintaining our weight. We need to do this forever.

This was my mother's first and foundational secret to living slim: she valued real food.

That isn't, however, the end of the story. We are not stopping and staying here. Because, my mum had more than one tool in her slim-living arsenal. And that is what we're going to discover next.

CHAPTER 3

Ever the Diplomat

The idea of emotional overeating has been a popular concept for some time; it was a concept utterly and completely foreign to my mother.

Emotional eating: yes. She relished her food as much as anyone.

Emotional overeating: no. Never.

My mother's home province, famous at home and abroad for its inhabitants' bluff good humour and generosity of spirit, is situated in the cold Atlantic waters off Canada's east coast. Her early life, in those perhaps more structured times, contained many rituals and celebrations that featured good and plentiful foods.

One food detail she referenced many a time, however, was that Newfoundland, in her time, did not have access to plentiful supplies of milk for children. Like the rest of Canada and all of North America, it certainly does now. In fact, its dairy processing industry is a steady and booming business.

But my mother often told me how tea – usually laced with

canned milk – was consumed early and regularly throughout a child's young life, rather than the steady supplies of fresh, whole milk she made sure we drank.

Other eating habits were also perhaps not the best. Newfoundland "hard tack" is an extremely hard, dried biscuit which was reconstituted by soaking in water for several hours and was therefore a useful provision, in days gone by, for sailors and fishermen far from home. It was made entirely of white flour however, devoid of the nutrients and any of the fibre of the whole grain; guaranteed not to go bad, but also guaranteed to be vitamin-free.

But, on the beautifully enjoyable other hand, tart, sweet, tangy berries were everywhere, in season. Fish was plentiful, of course. And most people lived a life that kept them closely in touch with the land and active living.

Even in a small city like St. John's, people often grew what they could either in backyard gardens or in land just outside the city. My mother's father – my grandfather – kept track of such activities in his journal noting the sowing of cabbage seeds in the spring and, on September 25, 1903, that his father had "set 700 strawberry plants in a new plot today."

My mum loved dandelion greens. They provided some of the first bright, little offerings of spring when she was young, and she consumed them, with much pleasure, throughout her life.

During all of my mother's early years, the families surrounding her had eating traditions that were frugal of necessity and that focused on food that sustained. A meal did not pass where gratitude was not expressed for the nourishment that was on the table and for the company in which it was consumed.

This closeness to the origins of our food supplies, their careful husbandry, as well as a sense of gratitude, celebration, and creativity when it comes to consuming meals have been common wherever and whenever we humans have lived.

One of the mainstays of life and nourishment for many First Nations peoples in Canada and other places in North America used to be the mighty and abundant acorn.

Now under consideration by the commercial food industry for its potential use in gluten-free products, this tidy little kernel could be carefully stored to last throughout the winter. It was ingeniously leached of its bitter tannic acid and then ground into an exceedingly nutritious flour, full of good oils and protein, more or less comparable to the nutritive value of almonds or hazelnuts.

Interestingly, the popular cashew, another highly nutritious tree nut, (native to Brazil and carried to the rest of the world by the Portuguese in the 1500s), is also carefully stripped of a bitter toxin before it enters our stores and kitchens.

In my mother's time, edible acorn meal and ready-to-eat cashews were not top of mind among her food choices. But, the same type of respect for valuable and sometimes scarce sources of nutrition, so common and essential throughout human existence, certainly permeated her own.

For example, in her time, it was common to use every last scrap of any meat that was consumed, including the "scrunchions" which were the leftover scraps of fat remaining from a roast of pork or beef. These scrunchions were fried up for their flavour but also for their helpful caloric value. They were used to enhance the content of later meals — much like bacon bits without the chemicals.

This was well before people began to worry about the impact on heart health of too much animal fat — a worry that now seems to be diminishing as differing viewpoints arise. But it was also a time when people walked a great deal, worked hard, and made use of those particular calories.

Throughout her life, my mother valued good, balanced, reasonably hearty, sit-down family meals and special treats for special occasions. It never crossed her mind to deprive herself of these occasional pleasures – including any available scrunchions.

But the operative word regarding any food extravagance was *occasional*. And her corresponding attitude was one of discipline.

In fact, she brought discipline to all her endeavours; much more so than I ever could or did. But this didn't, for a moment, mean that discipline trumped joy in her life. The concepts do not, each other, negate. Much as marketing campaigns might have us think that joy derives from more and more consumption, it simply doesn't. Joy derives from achievement, creation, creativity, usefulness, appreciation, and love, all of which my mother experienced in spades, and none of which made her heavier than she wanted to be.

I do know, however, that my mother loved her treats. And I readily admit that I likely inherited a good deal of my love of good food from her. Just as I seem to have inherited her affection for beautiful sunsets like the ones that stretched in glowing perfection over the agricultural dykelands that lay just beyond our Annapolis Valley home.

Fortunately for my mother, her definition of treats extended to a piece of fine steamed salmon or delicate fresh cod as well as layered servings of tender Swiss chard. I do believe she enjoyed these items as much any piece of homemade fruitcake at Christmas and far more than any fast food she occasionally allowed into her life.

But my mother did live in the 20th century. She did witness the modern rise and then explosion of commercially produced food products. She lived in a time and a place that saw many of us tempted not only by too much junk food but also by too much good food. She was not immune to advertising. And she definitely had to manage her taste for treats during a lifetime in which she never really ruled out any food type and while the world around her headed with fast-moving pace towards obesity.

Aside from valuing and prioritizing natural foods throughout her life, what other secret helped her manage these pressures and remain slim?

Well, it was another simple concept, really. My mother knew, in her bones, that while a small amount of a delightful thing is delightful, a too-large amount of the very same thing ruins the experience.

She knew that over-indulgence in even the best of food tires the senses and overloads the body. Far better to stop when you're ahead was her implicit assumption. And she had the innate discipline to carry this out.

This is the second key belief and practice that helped my mother live slim for a lifetime and that continues to help other Canadian women do the same.

We may understand the concept in our own individual way, and we definitely apply it in ways that match our personal tastes and circumstances, but this deeply important idea is critical in successfully managing slim and healthy lives in today's world.

It was a brilliant fall day when I shared a meal with my globe-trotting niece – one of my mother's slim grandchildren – on the busy, hilly, cobble-stoned Royal Mile in the charming City of Edinburgh, Scotland. People were walking up and down the narrow street, happily enjoying its historical significance – and its souvenir shops! Several small busloads of visiting adventurers had already made their way off the street and out of the city to explore castles, whisky distilleries and Scotland's magnificent mountains and coasts.

Together, my niece and I were taking a break from our respective explorations. The invigorating air of the September day and the old-but-new ambience of this ancient city formed a perfect backdrop to the thoroughly modern little eatery where we met. The place was packed with young people. Its specialty appeared to be super-fresh food of the healthier variety and a tantalizing array of mixed salads. We made our choices. We found our seats. We chatted. We ate. People came and went through the open door. Our little round table was the perfect location to enjoy the action.

The servings were generous but I did, indeed, manage to polish off pretty well every last scrap on my plate. My young niece was not quite so determined. As our meal wound to a close, she announced herself full and finished – with a significant portion of remnants still on her plate.

"But," she announced with her dazzling smile, "people should always eat just two-thirds of what's on their plate anyway."

I nodded. I did understand.

But, to myself, I also smiled. And I thought of my mother.

My slim and tiny mother. My niece's grandmother. My sensible, cost-conscious, Newfoundland-raised mother. She would have been well and truly shocked at such a statement. And, frankly, she would not have accepted it in silence either. To order food in a restaurant and then routinely, consciously "waste" one-third?

My mother's ongoing sense of frugality, born of the Depression, but, more important, also born of a lifetime of modest living, would have been profoundly disturbed.

But then my slim and tiny mother would also have been very hard-pressed to have consumed the portions served on our plates that day and the often over-large portions dished up by many restaurants in our time. In fact, I know she wouldn't have been able to finish it all, especially in her later years.

What this slender granddaughter was expressing – without realizing it – was really a kind of present-day update to her slim grandmother's own way of thinking.

In our time of plenty, with everyone eating out so much more frequently, with all of us surrounded by food that is not really food, eating just two-thirds of the often too-large servings we encounter is indeed one way of coping.

It is indeed one way – and not a bad one at that – of making a conscious and deliberate decision to avoid our current habit of over-eating and the excess weight gain that happens slowly, but surely, as a result.

Another of my mother's slim grandchildren, one of my own daughters, surveyed the array of food that filled our dining table not too long ago and expressed a virtually identical sentiment in another way: "Weight control is all about portion control," she said calmly, if a bit bluntly, as she helped herself to a little bit of everything on offer. "That's it. That's all. As far as I'm concerned, a person can eat anything they want. As long as their portions are okay."

All things, but all things in moderation, is how my mother might have put it. If she had spent any time at all even thinking about weight control!

The term "portion control" wasn't in my mother's lexicon. Eating two-thirds of a plate, for her, would have meant helping yourself to less at the table, since she rarely ate out, and "wasting" food at home would have been frowned upon. Literally!

But life in balance – neither overdoing it nor underdoing it – was an approach that permeated her character completely. And along that score, in regards to food, she would have been completely in sync with her 21st century granddaughters.

My little mother lived a life that fully celebrated traditions and the joys of food, family and good times. But she balanced it throughout with a continuing sense of disciplined moderation. For her, food was absolutely an important aspect of life. It was not, however, the dominant part.

This may have seemed easy and automatic in my mother's time, in my mother's busy life, and in the lives of other women of her era. I remember very few of her friends, sisters, aunts, or great-aunts as being particularly overweight despite the relentless escalation of junk food and commercially created food products during the 1950s and '60s. For one thing, in my memory, which may indeed be faulty, they seemed to be constantly busy! Far too busy to put on pounds!

I say that, instinctively, although pairing slimness with busyness is not a reliable axiom at all. Sometimes, our too-busy lives almost seem to favour over-eating – but more on that later.

To assume, however, that it was easy and automatic for my mother and her friends to stay slim too readily implies that it took no effort, or that theirs was such a different time that we can learn nothing from their approach. That would be a mistake.

Yes, my mother benefited from her own upbringing earlier in the 20th century when fast food was not a routine part of life and when virtually all meals, in daily life as she knew it, were eaten at home. But as well, the art of moderation was an art that she and other women of her time learned, fine-tuned and practiced over time. It's an art still very much available to all of us. We just have to take the time to think about it.

One silly little memory that I cherish concerns ice cream in my growing-up years at home. What we remember, and why, and with what elements of emotion and interpretation, is all a great mystery in our lives. But there it is. Stored in my memory and surrounded at this point in my life with much nostalgic love.

When my mother brought home ice cream to her family of five, she generally just brought one of those small, one-pint cardboard boxes that you opened completely, folding down the sides and cutting the ice cream into slices. For our family, that meant the ice cream was available for one meal and one meal only. Then it was finished. It wasn't always in the house or always available. In a way, it was portion control.

And this is a food product that most definitely needs not just portion control but control in general!

Yes, of course, the very first iced creams and sorbets created thousands of years ago by creative food innovators were reasonably healthy and certainly delicious combinations of fruits, sweeteners, shaved ice, cream, and some sort of thickener. But, ice cream, as we know it now, has strayed far indeed from those origins, and very far indeed from the completely occasional pattern of consumption early iced-treat consumers would have practiced.

Ice cream packed in large tubs is now always available, always well-supplied, in every supermarket in the country. It's a staple and popular food product that enjoys special promotional pricing on an almost weekly basis. Some now consider it to be a necessary part of their daily lives.

My mother was right to provide it with caution to her young brood.

I didn't follow her closely on this particular path. I usually purchased ice cream in the two-litre size, and often had more than one variety in the freezer when my own young brood was growing up.

But I did have the smarts to consciously apply her custom of planned scarcity to another food product: potato chips.

These fatty platforms for salt were not at all a part of my mother's cultural past, and I don't remember them being available in her home for us as children.

My siblings and I discovered them, of course, as teenagers. Living in our very real world of the North American 1950s and '60s, we avidly, eagerly, and devotedly added them to our consumption routine – along with the intoxicating distraction of commercially prepared dips. I, personally, became very fond of this combination.

But – all the food marketing pressures of the '50s and '60s notwithstanding – my solid and sensible mother would have no more thought of serving these items alongside a sandwich for lunch, as was promoted by the potato chip industry at the time, than she would have thought that a bowl of ice cream was an okay breakfast for her kids.

Let's take a moment to step back and think about that.

Because, did you know that positioning the potato chip as a food item to be served, not just for snacks but as part of a meal, was a planned strategic marketing tactic of the potato chip industry?

It's one really interesting example of the influence, ingenuity, and long-reaching impact of mid-century – and continuing – food marketing on our eating habits and consequent weight issues.

It is certainly true that ever since we humans have been around, we've devoted a great deal of effort to trying to understand exactly what compels us to do what.

But motivational psychology as an organized discipline – in fact psychology in general – was quite a bit of a new and evolving science in the early twentieth century. Trendy, even as it struggled to establish itself as a systematic discipline, it became widely used and extremely influential in the development of sales and marketing strategies.

Motivational psychologists worked for and with many advertising companies.

When they were hired by potato chip manufacturers to help them grow their sales, they determined, through surveys, analysis and deep thought, that many mid-century mothers – like my mother – viewed potato chips with some suspicion as a not-too-healthy snack item that should be consumed in moderation on special occasions only.

Sadly for the manufacturers of potato chips, this very intelligent view acted as a decided barrier to increased potato chip sales.

What to do? What to do? Sales of this new product were certainly huge, but they had reached a plateau. Things couldn't be left to stagnate like that.

Motivational psychologists soon came up with the answer: create a new image of the potato chip as a standard food item that could be consumed any old time in the most ordinary of circumstances, a food item that the caring, modern mother should really have in the kitchen cupboard every single day of the week.

The most effective way to do this, the motivational psychologists said, was to promote the use of potato chips in school cafeterias, other institutional eateries, as well as in restaurants and the average home as items to be served *on the plate* with other foods at mealtime. This would imply they were not just snacks, but legitimate accompaniments to normal meals. Caring, modern mothers would see this and draw the appropriate conclusions.

Glossy magazine advertising supported this effort with vigour. Homemakers viewed legions of grilled cheese sandwiches, with potato chips on the side, hundreds of hamburgers and fixings, with potato chips on the side, bowls and bowls of steaming soup, with potato chips on the side. Every lunch meal that North American children might possibly consume at school, in a restaurant, or at a backyard celebration was depicted, with potato chips on the side.

A second important tactic was also proposed by motivational psychologists: promote the use of potato chips as a substitute for real potatoes in home-style cooking.

Suddenly, mid-century moms were clipping out recipes for one-dish meals that called for not just tinned soups – which were everywhere at that time – but also for "two cups of crushed potato chips" as an easy and seemingly okay substitute for the real thing. An over-the-top dive into an ocean of salt if ever there was one!

Creating recipes that used commercial food products was an absolutely standard advertising tactic throughout this time, and remains a stunningly successful food marketing tool.

And again, the psychological objective of this far-reaching effort was to eliminate any distrust consumers had for this product and to replace that distrust with the idea that potato chips were a healthy food item that could be served frequently and confidently to children and families.

The twin-pronged strategy was wildly successful. Beyond the potato chip industry's most expansive expectations.

To this day, you'll still find potato chips served as "sides" in more than a few hospital cafeterias and even some restaurants. Granted, a bit of a retro image now – but actively embraced as such!

To this day, sales of potato chips worldwide are extremely high, currently accounting for about 35 percent of sales in the global savoury snack food market despite all kinds of changes in our understanding about the impact on our health of salt, fats, and processed foods in general!

Certainly, anywhere in Canada or the United States, a quick peek into any local convenience store confirms that a huge chunk of shelf space is always devoted to this product.

Full disclosure here: I have eaten my share of these items in my life. I became completely enamoured of them in my teens. And I was completely culturally attuned to them as the standard and indispensable party snack of my 1960s era.

However, and fortunately, I was health-conscious enough as a young adult and a young mother that, when my kids were young, I bought them only occasionally for special times.

Thinking about it now, I realize I was somewhat mimicking the discipline inherent in my mother's one-pint boxes of ice cream.

When potato chips of any variety were finished in my house of youngsters, they were finished. They were not an item that was routinely available. They were never added to my list of staples for grocery shopping. They were never, ever served with meals.

I did, quite often, bring home a bag of corn chips hoping, perhaps vainly, that they represented a somewhat healthier variation. And my kids did, quite happily, consume those corn chips with salsas and homemade yogurt dips for years, until teenage-hood set in, when they forged their own paths through a junk-food world, before looping back to outstandingly good choices in adulthood.

But, enough about motivational psychology and that saga of salt.

Let's turn our thoughts to another immensely popular food product. One that my mother did indeed love. That would be chocolate. It's amazing, when you think about it: this weird, firm mixture of exceedingly bitter brown beans ground up and mixed with fat and sugar. And we all seem to love it.

In fact, we seem to be consistently helpless when confronted with certain stimulating, often-bitter, chemical compounds that crop up in our teas, our coffees, and chocolates.

But in this case, too, my mother practiced moderation. I distinctly remember her enjoying this treat, but when she did occasionally indulge herself, she brought home some chocolate for the family, had a few pieces herself, and shared the rest. It was never routinely available for snacking.

She sounds like the perfect model of restraint, doesn't she? Well, she did grow up in an age and environment – and in a family – where restraint was expected, necessary, and normal. And maybe there is something to reflect on there.

I will admit, however, that as a teenager, I was not nearly so restrained. I knew well where she kept all of her baking supplies. Including those tempting, half-used and refolded packages of chocolate chips.

And I also knew well the guilty pleasure of just-a-few and just-a-few-more stolen bites raided from her pantry shelves.

And, as an aside, yes, they were very real, down-home, pantry shelves.

Our pantry was the absolutely cutest little room at the back of the house, tucked behind both the kitchen and the adjacent dining room. It had a window even, looking out onto the backyard, and two doors: one that entered from the kitchen, the other that opened onto the dining room. It had a wooden counter – truly, all wood, no laminate or marble finish at all – and wooden shelves, as well as steps that marched up to the ceiling and ended there, on which we piled assorted foods. High in one corner, on a small, triangular shelf, was my mother's sewing basket.

Not to linger in the memory of that pantry too long, the point remains that whether it was ice cream, chips, or chocolate, my mother consistently practiced the careful art of moderation as she managed her life and raised her family.

But she had another ace up her sleeve as well: the somewhat more delicate art of diplomatic refusal.

When offered cookies, candies, or other sweets while visiting other people's homes or eating out anywhere, she took one, perhaps two, and then gently turned aside the rest.

Her word for anything extra sweet or extra fatty was "rich."

"My, that was a rich meal," she might say in her later years. "It was delicious," she'd be quick to add, ever the diplomat, "but I won't have that dessert now, thank-you. I'll have some a bit later."

Not for my mother either gobbling or secret eating. She ruled her food. To my knowledge, food never ruled her.

I wasn't quite so lucky. Perhaps it was the more indulgent era in which I grew up. Perhaps it was the plenty that surrounded me and the easy access to store-bought treats that started with the earliest small bits of weekly allowance that burned a hole in my pocket. Perhaps it was just my temperament.

But I'm sure, as well, that it was the constant and overwhelming promotion and advertising of food products that permeates all aspects of our modern culture and that certainly permeated my formative years in the ′50s and ′60s.

We've all lived and breathed and absorbed this advertising for so many years that we can barely conceive of a world that isn't constantly bombarded with messages to eat – and generally to eat something that is cheaply made with large quantities of fat, sugar, starch and salt.

Actually, we can barely conceive of a world without advertising, period.

Whatever the reason, starting in my late teens, I began to

over-indulge in items that were sweet, salty, fatty, or sour.

Learning the lesson of moderation did not happen automatically. It actually took almost a lifetime. As a matter of fact, certain techniques of moderation didn't even enter my daily life until I was over fifty when I discovered my metabolism had slowed to something resembling a lazy crawl, and I began to gain weight even without the dubious pleasure of over-indulgence! More on that later.

But for Canadian women who adopt the approach of moderation, planned scarcity and diplomatic refusal early in their lives – perhaps as a natural outcome of their temperaments, perhaps as a conscious choice – slim, trim living is easy and very pleasurable indeed. What's not to like, after all? None of your favourite foods is off limits!

Some women, like my globe-trotting young niece, might decide to limit themselves to eating only two-thirds of what's on their plate when eating out. Others might decide to use smallish dinner plates and fill them with smaller portions accordingly. Others may choose to enjoy a dessert at home just once a week, making it, therefore, an especially special occasion.

I was a young mother living in Mississauga, just outside Toronto, when community work brought me in touch with Sofia. Some twenty-five years my senior, her children grown and independent, she was living very comfortably when I met her, enjoying her work, and giving time to community projects.

One day she told me, with a smile of fond remembrance, about her younger years with little children. Living on a tight budget, she and her husband used to splash out a bit on Fridays. That evening, they would always indulge in a dessert – a purchased apple pie.

So simple, so ordinary, I remember thinking. Fruit pies were readily available and fairly inexpensive in our country then and now. But that was their celebration, their shared reward at the end of a busy week, and a memory that she still held, sweet and cherished, in her mind.

It was also an experience of enjoyable moderation because the rest of their week was dessert-free.

We did not evolve under conditions of unrelenting plenty as regards to food supply. We evolved searching for food, episodically going long periods with little food, eating well of natural things when we found them, and getting along without much when we had to. Episodes of food scarcity have been completely natural in our evolutionary history and our bodies understand them well. Planned scarcity in our modern lives of over-flowing food abundance — that is to say an ongoing approach of moderation — is something our bodies can handle much better than ongoing over-indulgence.

Taking our worldview out of the animal kingdom just for a moment: have you ever seen an overweight tree? Trees have many of the basic life-supporting needs that we have. They need food. They need water. Their circulatory system is remarkably like our own. But they always take up only what they need. They have ways of conserving energy for times of drought and cold and fire. But in times of plenty — lots of water, no cold, no fire — they certainly flourish, propagate, grow tall, diversify, create forests of themselves, but they still do not become unhealthily overweight.

But that's the vegetable kingdom.

In contrast, our flexible, malleable, wonderful but convoluted human brain has taken us in quite a different direction indeed. And, as some of that direction relates to food and its over-consumption, we now have to consciously apply the intelligence of our malleable brains to the situation.

So, let's think about it. Let's think about our own unique particulars.

Let's think about very good sweet treats occasionally, but small in size. Nuts because they're wonderful and good for us, but not by the cupful and perhaps not salted as that salty taste stimulates us to eat beyond our natural appetite. Cheese, especially good ones, but in small delectable pieces, not great gobs, and definitely not slathered on everything like a sauce. Ice cream in small dishes, savoured slowly, not three-scoop cones.

Let's think about good breakfasts, lunches and dinners, but little in between except fruits, vegetables, a quiet cup of tea or long drinks of cooling water.

As for juice and pop, I'd say never. Pop is sugar water and chemicals, period. Juices may have a modicum of value, but it's just a modicum, and they can set us up for the unhealthy reliance on the sugar rush of sweetened soft drinks almost as much as the soft drinks themselves.

The approach of moderation means choosing what we'll eat, when we'll eat it, and what trade-offs we'll make if and when we know we've overdone it. It means consciously, slowly, and deliberately integrating our intelligence with our emotions and our drives.

Let's sit with that thought for a moment: what we'll eat, when we'll eat it, and what trade-offs we'll make if and when we know we've overdone it.

This is a positive thing, not a negative.

This does *not* mean giving up all the delicious treats and food experiences that are so much a part of our personal cultural heritages.

But this does mean it may take time and some conscious self-talk for some of us to land in a place of acceptance.

Some of the better restaurants in Canada – and not necessarily expensive ones – are now, fortunately, becoming better versed in the art of smaller servings.

I have enjoyed just-right portions of fresh-seared scallops and simple, but oh-so-delicious, home-cooked vegetables in a roadside diner in rural Nova Scotia, all the while losing myself to the tall, unclipped sway of grasses blown by the wind across the road.

I have lingered over wonderfully seasoned shrimp and sole steamed in a banana leaf in an unassuming eatery filled with quiet voices and classical music along a gritty section of Toronto's Danforth Avenue.

And I have had the privilege of watching the temporarily peaceful but incredibly powerful movements of the Bow River in Alberta as I was served a delicious and perfectly sized salad in the grand old hotel that dominates the town of Banff.

I recently enjoyed the new-to-me and totally captivating flavours of an Algerian salad: a just-right serving of ground beans and vegetables with tuna and olives – yum – in a small jot of an eatery on a busy Toronto street.

As for memories of our succulent Canadian lobster, if I *had* to choose, it would be that small riverside location in Prince Edward Island, where sun danced on shimmering water and all seemed well with the world as I enjoyed a delicious and perfectly proportioned meal.

(But if I didn't have to choose, I'd rave on about the perfect, waterfront freshness of Hall's Harbour lobster on Nova Scotia's Fundy shore, and the fabulous, one-of-a-kind lobster roll at Wolfville's Blomidon Inn!)

Such wonderful, fresh and satisfying food actually encourages us not to over-do as every mouthful is good and good for us.

I'm grateful for the choice we're now offered of smaller and better portions, but this approach is far from universal. Not every restaurant presents its food already plated. I'm thinking here of buffets.

Long and accurately burdened with the reputation of laden plates and indiscriminate overeating, buffets can be a challenge even as they are immensely popular in our country.

But some of my most delightful meals have been at buffet tables. One must simply – although yes, with some difficulty – choose with discernment.

One of my most memorable buffet meals took place on the ferry boat connecting Vancouver with Victoria in our west coast province of British Columbia. I wasn't expecting it, which is perhaps what made the experience that much more enjoyable. I've traversed waters on all kinds of ferry boats in my life, and most did not feature fine dining. Quite the opposite, I'd say.

This boat, however, advertised a buffet lunch, and my husband and I observed that people were quickly and eagerly lining up for it. Must be good, we thought cautiously. Although on a ferry boat? Really??

Well, it was a fabulous spread. All kinds of good things from soup, to salad, to dessert. And, perhaps it was just the day, but both my husband and I swear it was the best steamed salmon we've ever tasted before or since. It was one of those times when you're tempted to overeat. But again, my mother's wisdom: a little bit of a wonderful thing is wonderful, too much tires the senses.

We ate slowly, savouring the items we had chosen; the whole experience enhanced by our passing view of the beautiful waters, blue sky, and treed islands, both distant and near.

One of my favourite places here in Toronto is a large, very popular Middle Eastern buffet. Yes, one could easily overdo it.

But with a dose of respect for oneself and a nod to moderation, one could also enjoy a perfectly sized plate of grilled eggplant, creamy hummus, tangy tabouli, scented beets, delicately seasoned chicken liver, grilled cauliflower, oven-fresh bread and more. All without feeling overwhelmed.

Even Canada's all-day breakfast – still our national deal-on-wheels – is changing and evolving.

You'll rarely find the "full English" version, with its servings of beans and fried tomatoes. But for generations, Canadians have consumed eggs fried, poached, or scrambled, with bacon, sausage, or ham, a whole cartload of hash browned potatoes, plus toast with butter and jam. An unapologetic plateful of very sustaining protein, fat and carbohydrate, at a very good price.

But now, it's being lightened and brightened all over the place.

In my experience, it was Montreal's lively neighbourhood cafés that took the Canadian lead on this. But, you can now find lashings of fruit and mountains of greens bumping into over-easy eggs in hole-in-the-wall student eateries in downtown Toronto, and increasingly innovative breakfasts and brunches everywhere.

I've personally become fond of the offering that I first sampled in Australia and that is now broadly available here: mashed avocado on wholegrain toast topped with delicate poached eggs and a light sprinkle of, perhaps, chili-garlic oil or sumac. Delicious! I now also make it at home.

Of course, you can always request a lighter version of breakfast just about anywhere. Simple poached egg on toast is certainly the all-day-breakfast friend of many a Canadian woman over fifty.

For all of us, in fact, there is a compromise and a lighter/healthier adjustment to just about every food we associate with our pleasurable activities. What we have to do is make the effort to imagine it, to try it out, and to be willing to give it the same amount of time to become part of our lives as we've allowed for other less valuable – and more weight-inducing – habits to develop.

If we can have one piece of blueberry pie but not have two, we're practicing moderation. If we can enjoy that lovely plate of latkes but go easy on the dessert, we're doing well. If we can top our coffee with cream but regulate how many coffees we regularly consume, more power to us.

And, if we can relish every single bite of those flat-out amazing eggs Benedict, served over warm, crunchy fishcakes in the busy gastro-pub near my Annapolis Valley hometown – but, *big* but – follow that up with very light later indulgences, we are certainly enjoying the best of all possible worlds.

Now, if we can just convince our families to watch Hockey Night in Canada without the chips and dip.

Well. Sigh. Okay. Maybe some things are a bit more difficult.

Perhaps we can allow the less-than-healthy habits one Saturday night and a plateful of beautiful fruits and vegetables the next! Nothing ventured, nothing gained, as my dear mother might have said. For all of my family, homemade, fresh-popped popcorn has been a saving grace in these circumstances.

In terms of my personal food weakness, I may as well admit that I'm a devoted browser of pastry shops wherever I happen to go. But, here's my compromise: browsing doesn't always mean buying.

I'm quite sure that pastry shop owners don't think of their places as a sort of museum for the viewing. But in my strange little way, I do.

Having said that, my bones do tell me that life is short and some food creations must simply be enjoyed in the moment.

I have been known to have a really over-the-top dessert (think sticky toffee pudding, with ice cream, in a British pub) and just call that lunch: done and done.

Okay. Here's the back story. I was on a trip through the British Isles where sticky toffee pudding had been offered quite a few times on the menu following a regular meal. Each time, I was too full from the regular meal to have a dessert. But, the sticky toffee pudding looked wonderful and kept calling and calling. Finally, I just had to answer the call with a full-on lunch effort devoted solely to it. And it was totally worth it!

Some slim Canadian women routinely make a next day effort to cut back after indulging in meals that may have featured plentiful wine or any other kind of fulsome splurge.

When our appetites and metabolisms are in balance, this is a completely natural tendency. The body instinctively wants to rest a bit or make a change after any over-indulgence whether that be too much food, too much work, too much play – or even too much solitude.

Equilibrium, however attained, is fundamental to our functioning. It is fundamental to life itself. And it is something we instinctively recognize as good if we take the time and create the silence to let this awareness take hold.

When our appetites and metabolisms are out of balance, however, when we've essentially lost touch with the signals our own bodies send us, then we have to consciously embrace and practice this habit of counter-balance, this natural gravitation toward equilibrium.

The first time I came across this concept was the same time that I discovered the joys of English trifle in a pleasant home in the town of Sherbrooke in Quebec's Eastern Townships – *les Cantons de l'Est*. The area is one of Canada's many beautiful agricultural regions and is located just east of Montreal.

I worked at a summer camp in the region for three happy years as a teenager, and I visited this home with one of my co-workers during that time.

Granted the English trifle I tasted – and took the recipe for – was not quite the traditional mixture. Like many a recipe that went through the mill of the corporate food industry in the 1950s and '60s, it called for brand-name products. Not a drop of sweet sherry in this one. Rather, it required a particular type of packaged jelly mix. And the vanilla custard was not made from scratch with egg yolks as thickener, but used a ready-made mix in which yellow dye gave the appearance of eggs.

Despite that, the end result was really very delicious to my young tastes, featuring thin slices of buttery pound cake (not ladyfingers), bananas, sliced, tinned pears, the vanilla custard, raspberry jelly, and freshly whipped cream. I was utterly hooked. I knew that the recipe, written out on a little index card that I still retain, would travel back with me to my Annapolis Valley home. And I knew it would soon be shoe-horned into our family dessert traditions.

However, I was 18 at the time, already aware that I was inclined to overdo it when it came to food consumption, and already starting to gain a few excess pounds. I recall talking through my thoughts with my friend whose mother had made the dessert.

"How does your mum make these things, and eat these things, and still stay slim?" I asked her. For her mum was an extremely trim-looking woman in her forties at the time who looked in calm control of her life to my 18-year-old eyes.

"She cuts back the next day," said my friend. "She's done that for years. She could easily gain weight. She's told me that. But she has this habit where, the very day after she has a dessert like this, she just always cuts back. She says it's easier to do it right away than to let it pile up."

For whatever reason, I hadn't quite thought of things that way before.

I was already obsessing quite a bit too much over a few pounds gained here and there. I was also weighing myself too frequently, which was becoming a discouraging and somewhat compulsive habit. And my life was firmly affected by thoughts and experiments with drastic, oh-how-will-I-ever-summon-the-willpower types of diets.

I'd never really thought that one could overdo it a bit one day, and simply, calmly, quietly, and with no fuss whatsoever, cut back a bit the next.

The memory of this concept has stayed with me ever since.

I admit I could not and did not fully embrace such a quietly disciplined approach in my early years. But it lodged stubbornly in my mind as an idealized goal. And, amazingly, over the long haul, it became one of the foundational components of my personal approach to weight control.

It was only in recent years, however, that I came to realize how very instinctual this approach can be if we slow down and pay attention to how we interact with food.

I never had a conversation like that with my own slim mother. In fact, I never had a conversation with my own slim mother about weight control at all. So, I don't really know if she consciously cut back after overeating. I rather suspect that she did feel that instinctive take-a-break sensation that we experience if our appetites have not become too terribly disordered. I certainly know that she ate in moderation most of the time – a little bit of everything and nothing to excess. And I know, for sure, that it worked.

But no matter how we manage it – ongoing moderation, eating two-thirds of a plate, careful diplomacy, planned scarcity, portion control, prompt cutting back – the great and outstanding benefit of this balanced and moderate approach to eating is that we don't really rule anything out of our diet. We end up with access to all the amazing and ingenious things people do with food, as well as all the multitudinous nutrients that we seem to need to keep our bodies ticking.

We allow ourselves to enjoy anything we happen to enjoy – but we don't allow ourselves to enjoy it to excess. We choose and we decide. We balance as we go. And preferably, we balance quite soon after any overindulgence.

We've had a larger lunch than usual? We take a break and just have soup or salad for dinner tonight.

We've gone a bit overboard on wine one evening? The next day, it's simply yogurt and fruit for lunch.

With this approach, there is no feeling of pressing hardship that comes from thinking that we can't have this or can't have that in our daily diet or, conversely, that we can *only* have this or *only* have that. And we gain a nice sense of control over our life and our food.

Moderation in all things, however we understand it, is the second major tactic that kept my own mum slim, and that is useful, necessary, and still much practiced by Canadian women successfully living slim in our era of over-flowing plenty.

But, there is a major caveat to this approach.

While it works for many women, it does not work for some. The next chapter deals with the not-so-uncommon exception to the rule. It will reveal, as well, the third key factor that can make or break the efforts of some Canadian women as they endeavour to live slim.

CHAPTER 4

Adrianna's Choice

She was a woman with a delightful personality. Kind, gentle, always a good word for others. Dark hair framing a full face. Dark eyes always showing a thoughtful interest in those around her. Adrianna was one of the nicest people I'd ever met.

And for years she carried, I'd say, about 100 extra pounds. I'd never known her slim.

Her weight just seemed a part of who she was. She never mentioned it. Never indicated it bothered her. And it never dawned on me she might want to lose it. That's just how it was.

While we were work colleagues, we were not in the same department and didn't work closely together. But we chit-chatted now and then, whenever our paths would cross.

At one time, our departments were located near each other. Then we moved. And in our larger premises, our paths crossed much less frequently.

Then, one year, it must have been nine or ten months – perhaps more – since I'd seen her. And when I did, I did a literal double take.

It was morning and I was heading in to work, already consumed with thoughts of the day ahead. As I pushed through the large, double glass doors of the building, another staff member happened to be coming along just behind me. With my hand still holding the door, I gave an automatic glance backwards and caught sight of the woman approaching.

She seemed somewhat familiar, but very vaguely so. Something about the eyes. She reminded me of someone. She reminded me of... Adrianna! And she was smiling at me. And her smile was like Adrianna's. But this tall, slim woman coming through the doors couldn't possibly be Adrianna. Definitely not. Surely not.

That's when I did the literal and somewhat embarrassing double-take.

I had returned her smile politely, turned to continue inside, reconsidered, turned back, and stared.

"Adrianna?" I queried.

She smiled even more broadly.

"Oh. My. Goodness!"

As we both stepped away from the incoming foot traffic and found space at one side of the large, inner foyer, I realized there could be no dancing around this one. Those 100 pounds were gone. *Completely gone.*

It must have been months, I realized, since I'd seen her. And if I had seen her during the early weeks of weight loss, I suppose I wouldn't have noticed. But now it was all gone.

Mission. Completely. Accomplished.

Of course we all know that dramatic weight loss is famously hard to maintain. So, even then, I silently hoped for the best for her. But, regardless, in that precise moment, I was simply bowled over. Couldn't believe it at all. She looked great, and, ever gracious, she accepted my congratulations and best wishes.

"How did you do it?" I asked.

"You know, Lillian, it really wasn't anything special," she said. "This isn't rocket science. We all know what we have to do. I just ate less. I ate healthy stuff. I did what everyone tells you to do. I cut out the junk. I went for a walk every day. That's what I did. But, do you know what else I really, really had to do?"

I looked at her expectantly.

"I had to stop going into the bread section of the store. Yeah, completely," she said with a smile, as my face registered blank surprise. "Bread is my big weakness. Always has been. So I stayed out of the bread section of my grocery store completely. Completely. That's what I did."

"Wow," was all I could really muster, her comments necessarily repeating in the face of my complete astonishment.

We did chat some more of course, once I'd slightly recovered. Because I was curious. I'd never heard a comment like that in my life. Bread as her great nemesis? That ordinary plain-Jane of foodstuffs? So simple, so basic, so unassuming?

It wasn't that she had eliminated all starch, she clarified. Nor was she on any form of a high-protein diet. She didn't find potatoes addictive, or pasta, or other starches. She didn't avoid those during her year of weight loss. But with bread it was all or nothing, she said. She knew herself well enough to know. So, she made her choice.

I was bowled over.

I had never really thought of the bread departments of our everyday Canadian supermarkets as exuding quite that kind of siren call, exerting quite that degree of influence that someone would have to physically avoid them in order to stick with a weight loss plan.

Yes, I also love bread. Yes, I also love it with butter. And yes, I can still enjoy few things more than the first bite into a dense, chewy, well-made slice of leavened heaven.

But, if anything, I would have thought something sweeter, fattier or saltier would have been the demon monster in her closet, luring her off the beaten path of living slim: perhaps too many restaurant meals; too many bottles of wine; too many slices of tiramisu; or too many cherry chocolates hidden in the basement freezer in hopes you wouldn't eat them all at once.

But no. It was just bread, pure and simple.

Clearly, one person's plain-Jane, everyday food item can be an almost insurmountable obstacle in the path of somebody else.

Adrianna's strength was knowing this full-on and deciding to manage this particular weakness in a way that worked for her within her otherwise completely ordinary weight-loss regime. It was a true and thoroughly personal thought process at work.

As to why at midlife – she was then in her mid-forties – she chose to make the change?

Several health situations had recently affected her close family, she said. Serious health issues with evident links to excess weight. And while she, herself, did not have children to consider, these situations involving her siblings had caused her to look mortality in the face. She'd decided to act.

I left her that day, expressing my congratulations and support for her extraordinary effort, and believing, as well, that this was not a temporary diet but a life change for Adrianna.

I'm thrilled to add that, many years later, she is still as slim as she was that day, although I don't actually know if she ever allowed herself to step back into the bread department.

This is the third key insight and concept that can, if we let it, offer vital support for Canadian women who are trying to live slim.

If we know there is a food or a food habit in our lives over which we have no control, we can find the strength to face this fact and deal with it knowing it will make or break any effort to lose or control our weight.

If this food or food habit has become an addictive force in our lives then we need to decide whether we can have it in our lives, or whether we have to set it aside completely. We have to decide which is more important, this food and this habit, or our weight and health.

While Adrianna told me her story simply and honestly, it can be embarrassing to admit that we have eating habits, or any habits, that are out of control. Most of us would rather not admit it. And we'd also rather keep on indulging those habits. After all, we think they are enjoyable. We think they are soothing. We think they simply taste good. We think they make us happy. We may also think they take our minds off whatever discomfort or discontent is eating away at our psyches.

But like any addictive over-indulgence, these habits have a way of taking over.

Who knows by what deep neural mechanism they manage to do this, but they do. And who cares just why or how they started, they are there. We could waste a lot of time speculating, and we could waste this time with a box of chocolates or a bowl of ice cream at our side. The simple truth is these disordered habits never serve us well over the long haul.

Adrianna's choice – and Adrianna's strength – was to acknowledge this weakest link in her chain of resolve, face it down, and deal with it in a way that worked *for her.*

It's an option open to any woman who knows, deep down,

she has the same problem.

I don't know what my mother might have said to Adrianna, or thought of her choice.

I believe she might have found it hard to believe that any particular food could exert such a hold over someone. My mother had nothing even close to an addictive temperament. She undoubtedly felt anxiety, self-doubt, fear, sadness, regret, and all the other exhausting emotions that can pull us down and make us want to boost ourselves up with the help of a temporary, feel-good crutch. Her nature and her way of life, however, did not incline her to over-indulgence in order to accomplish this.

I, however, have a bit of Adrianna's problem. Many of us do. If not always with bread.

For me, it has often been chocolate, almost any kind of pie, and cashews.

I admit that for many, many years I was very weak when it came to good chocolate. Even inferior chocolate, if I'm completely honest.

For a while, I thought I would have to give up chocolate completely, as I could never seem to take just one piece. As long as a chocolate bar was in the house somewhere, it called out to me to finish it. One piece invariably became eight.

For long periods of time, I have used Adrianna's method: not tasting, not trying, not buying anything with chocolate.

Then I would try it and the old pull – the inclination to over-indulge – would return.

It's beyond my area of competence to dig deeply into the nature of addiction. It's sufficient for me to know that it does exist widely among us humans.

Some might think: Food addiction, oh, come on, what's the big deal? Not nearly as worrisome as gambling, drinking, doing drugs, etc. How can anyone possibly have a problem controlling their intake of certain kinds of food?

That would be how my husband would see it. He's never felt the pull to over-indulge with food. He routinely stops eating when he's full, even when the food is something he absolutely enjoys.

When I first met him, I was fascinated by the fact that he regularly stopped eating midway through a meal, seemingly to rest for a while before finishing. Many a time he would never finish! He is, in fact, a died-in-the-wool food dragger-outer: one who will never eat an entire, individual sour-cherry tart in one sitting; one who will save that last small piece of chocolate for seven days and then forget he has it; one who is loath to consume the last morsel of cheese in the fridge, often letting it dry to an inedible crust instead. He is the complete opposite of an addictive eater.

But, that's him. Then there's the rest of us.

Chocolate, we know, has certain stimulants, tons of fat, and varying amounts of sugar. And it seems to be a weakness for many.

But I have to wonder why cashews have also had this effect on me. Not almonds, hazelnuts, or walnuts – just cashews. And, to be clear, this is not roasted, salted cashews I'm talking about. I do understand that salt provides a particular kick all of its own. No, it's the raw, unroasted cashews that are on my list of foods I can't seem to resist.

And then pies. Again, why? All I can say is there's something about the crispy, flaky crust and the tart/sweet fruit filling of a well-made pie. One serving has never seemed to be enough.

One friend has told me that, despite the many health benefits of all kinds of nuts, she cannot keep any of them in the house as she finds she can never consume them in moderation. On the other hand, Nadeeka is able, unlike me, to happily enjoy just one piece of dark chocolate virtually every day after lunch and not be tempted to have more.

I have even wondered if for some people it is not the type of food that they find addictive, but the quantity. Perhaps very large servings provide some kind of satiated feeling that smaller servings do not.

As for Adrianna, the choice was clear: in order to take charge of her health, it was all or nothing for the bread. She chose health, and ditched the bread. I say more power to her and more power to any woman who engages in that sort of self-evaluation.

I must also say that quite often when I walk past the bread department in my local supermarket, I smile and think of her. I wonder if any of the staff busily filling shelves and tidying displays ever dreams that this most ordinary of departments could exert such bewitching power.

While I may smile at the thought, I do believe that this particular aspect of weight management is a serious one. Addictive and compulsive eating is real. It's common. And it's a challenge to address.

It was not an issue for my mother. She was lucky that way.

But, facing it down, as did Adrianna, is the third important element for some women in their efforts to live slim. A deal breaker, as some might say.

Up next: the fourth and final broad-brush concept related to living slim. It's one that I did, absolutely, learn from my mother, and one she would have been astonished to see included here.

CHAPTER 5

The Tea Ceremony

Tea was everywhere when I was growing up. My mother never understood how I could not – as a young adult and later as a mature adult – develop a taste for tea.

"You don't like tea yet?" she would say, for years, during visits to my home. *Yet* being the operative word.

It was inconceivable to her that I would not, at some point, come to my senses and appreciate tea.

Well, I never have. I'm a coffee person. I relish my cup of bitter delight first thing in the morning as much as she did hers – but it isn't tea.

Nowadays, we can debate the merits of green tea, black tea, chai tea, and a whole crateload of other varieties. But in my mother's house, it was your basic orange pekoe. Made with fresh water, just boiled, steeped just so, with milk, never cream, and a small jot of sugar to taste. She didn't do herbal, although, in later years, she kept a few such varieties on hand for visitors.

Coffee, on the other hand, was mainly your basic, nondescript, instant variety in my mother's home. A percolator did exist some-where in the back corners of her kitchen storage, but I swear I never saw it in use. My brother maintains that yes, he does have that memory. So, there may well have been some coffee-re-lated activities that I've forgotten. But, for sure, drip machines, filtered coffee, and all the many supports for our coffee-making endeavours were just beginning to enter the North American market at that time, and they never made a dent in my mother's tea-focused life.

Tea being so common in my upbringing, I remember wonder-ing, when I first heard about the Japanese tea ceremony, how anyone could make a ceremony of something people did every day. Wasn't it a bit like brushing your teeth or setting the table for dinner? Too commonplace for ceremony?

But then, one day, I stood in a small, wooden-roofed shelter in the exquisitely designed gardens of Toronto's Japanese Canadian Cultural Centre. Drifting greenery spread around me in all direc-tions. There was a blue sky overhead and an almost palpable quiet everywhere despite the fact that cars moved in unceasing rhythm along one of Toronto's endless, congested highways just over a treed embankment. I stood there. And I read a plaque that explained the custom. And somehow it all came clear.

Yes, it was a simple cup of tea, but yes, it was also so much more.

It was a ritualized quieting of the senses, an attention to detail, an acute experience of the particular that enabled a connection to the whole.

I understood it then as a moment of knowing that you are amazingly, incredibly, against-all-odds alive – and paying attention to that fact.

Although the term wasn't in my vocabulary at that time,

that was perhaps my first *gestalt* understanding of the concept of mindfulness.

And I thought of my mother.

In all my many years of knowing her, I never once saw my mother drink her cup of tea standing.

Nor did she drink it just before, or while in the process of, scooting off to somewhere or something else. And she was often scooting off to somewhere or something else.

And, most particularly, it was completely unheard of at that time for her, or anyone else, to walk down the streets of our small Annapolis Valley town gulping take-out tea, coffee, or anything else while also texting, talking, or rushing to work.

No.

Her cup of tea meant a moment of relaxation, in her own home. She would sit back in her chair, often physically exhaling a sigh. And her world would stop, temporarily, as she allowed herself to savour the flavour, as well as the mild lift it gave her.

It seemed a moment of repose – of thoughtfulness even – in the midst of her very active, always-busy life. Almost an excuse, or a reason, to stop and smell the roses, before resuming whatever tasks were at hand.

And I wonder if it is not these moments of pause, these interludes of quiet contemplation, these episodes of deliberate and somewhat ritualized "ceremony" that some of us now miss in our daily lives. I also wonder if sometimes we don't fill that void with the shallow solace of unnecessary food.

I had lunch in a busy, downtown Toronto dining room recently, during a busy, downtown Toronto working day. It was fall. The air was crisp and refreshing and there was a lovely breeze as I made my way across the wide expanse of public space in front of the curved-shell towers of our city hall.

The restaurant was one that routinely draws many lawyers because of its location near the central courthouse and also because of its excellent food.

As my lunch-mate and I settled in to our soups, in blew two young, black-gowned, women lawyers, deep in thought and conversation, heads down, footsteps hurried, as they headed for a nearby table.

I noticed them, especially, as they were close in age to my own daughters and reminded me of them. Each ordered quickly and then proceeded to spend the entire lunch consulting their phones, eyes barely lifting to the table, let alone to each other, let alone to the servers, let alone to the food. The working lunch refined and re-defined. I felt sorry for the unappreciated food. I felt more sorry for the two of them.

Hopefully, at some moment in their days and lives, they do take a moment to lift their eyes from their busyness, to acknowledge simple things, and to know that they are alive.

My mother was well familiar with busyness.

Canadian women of her generation and of her middle-class social and economic status did not, by any means, live in a soft-focus world of cut flowers in vases or idle afternoons.

She worked hard as a teacher in Newfoundland before she became a wife and a mother. I heard stories of those large classes. Forty boys, one year, remained in her memory as a particular challenge! She was a hands-on homemaker when she was a stay-at-home mum. She worked again as a teacher when she was widowed much too early. And she devoted considerable time throughout her life to her interests, her friends, her family and community endeavours.

She was a woman of active intelligence who did not collapse easily into nothingness or tranquility. In fact, she was frequently too busy, too studious, and too diligent for her own good. She had a bit of a hurried personality that was not entirely distant or different from the hurried distraction of the black-robed lawyers lunching near me in Toronto.

If she'd been born in their era, she might have been one of them, for she was a reasonably high achiever for her time and in her way. The recipient of much early coaching from a great-aunt, my mother did exceptionally well at school; she skipped two years in the early grades and then graduated, as a very young woman, from university in the 1930s when this was still quite rare for women in our country.

So yes, she knew all about busyness and hard work – as she also knew about unexpected loss and devastating heartbreak – but my busy and active mother did indeed relax with her tea.

She relaxed, as well, during certain other moments of particular calm and comfort: witnessing the appearance of those golden-red sunsets streaking across the western sky in the evening; understanding that her backyard garden was producing some excellent green beans; experiencing a particularly uplifting service at church; enjoying a piece of classical music on her kitchen radio.

Very basic, you say, but these were some of the moments that calmed her nerves, pulled her to a halt, kept her centred and connected to something quiet, private and elemental within herself. Something that I, as her daughter, could not truly know. Something that each one of us, as adults, keeps within us.

We all need those moments. And never more so than now, in our time of hurried everything: when cellphones are never off; when work invades every hour of our week; and when we live, very often, completely out of touch with the calming effects of nature.

Unfortunately for Canadian women, for North American women, and for women everywhere, snack food marketers know all too well how rushed, how frantic, and how disconnected many of us are from any sense of inner quiet in our lives. And they have the answer: sugar, generally mixed with fat.

Unfortunately, far too many of us have accepted their recommendation.

I attended a market research group once for a well-known brand of chocolate bar. I'm not sure how I got on their contact list, but there I was.

It was a group made up entirely of women. Some ten or twelve of us. I'm afraid my presence was an utter waste of their money, as I just couldn't take it as seriously as the organizers would have hoped. But, it was interesting.

A young man posed the questions, and what he attempted to probe, almost exclusively, was the emotional reason or reasons that would make us reach for this particular chocolate bar as a mid-afternoon or mid-evening break from routine.

I don't believe they touched mid-morning. Perhaps even chocolate bar producers know they'd be pushing it too far to try to associate something of no nutritional value to the morning. But as I try to recall this, I wonder: did he, actually, ask us about an 11 o'clock break? I'm not sure.

I do remember the great effort that was expended on his multitude of escalating questions. Were we rewarding ourselves? Were we taking a break? Was it a small indulgence? How did price factor in? Did price factor in? Was quality a factor? How much was quality a factor? What about the smoothness of the bar? Were we rewarding ourselves? What were we rewarding ourselves for? What about the idea that this bar was almost entirely targeted at women? Did we see this brand as a luxury brand? Were we rewarding ourselves? Were we rewarding ourselves? Were we rewarding ourselves?

I came out of that session believing, if nothing else, that the ad people very much hoped they could market this chocolate bar as a personal reward in our otherwise unrewarded life. Reward for all the stresses we tolerate. Reward for all the difficult jobs we endure. Reward for whatever at all that ails us.

While I would be the first to champion the wonderful sensations and experiences of well-prepared food in our lives, we are complicated beings. In our world of unending plenty, rewards of sugar and fat all too easily become repetitive habits that no longer soothe, or reward, or help us deal with our stresses, but rather *add* weight, *add* stress, and prompt an escalating anxiety.

We might just be better off to take a careful look at our crowded lives and consider what kind of reward we might receive from our own personal, zero-calorie tea ceremony instead.

Some people take a moment of pause with hot water alone.

Hot water! I thought when I first encountered this practice among my work colleagues of Asian background. Why on earth?

But at one point in my life, not being a tea lover, and drinking but one cup of coffee a day, I tried it, and tried it again – and then found myself adopting this practice. And I found that there is indeed something soothing and elemental about a simple cup of hot water. It slows you down. It gives you pause. And, if you let it, it can also allow you to take a moment to consider how you are really feeling. It can be your tea ceremony.

I have come to believe that an important factor in our modern problem with weight and appetite is a learned habit of reliance on excessively sweet, fatty, and salty food to distract us from our real feelings, especially feelings of pressure. We use food to free our minds from the uncomfortable, nagging, inescapable burdens in our lives, the stress of deadlines, responsibilities, and things still undone.

While these food items do seem to temporarily alleviate these feelings of pressure, to temporarily reward us for suffering through whatever we feel we are suffering through, the downside is precisely the dependent habit that leads to needing more and more of these unhealthy and fattening items to achieve the same distracting result.

We all have the option to choose otherwise.

My mother's calm moments – her tea ceremonies – cost absolutely nothing and were simply little quiet times that grew naturally from her background, her traditions, and her temperament.

But many of us, living in our more frantic age, may have to give some focused thought to creating these soothing moments in our lives.

Many Canadian women have adopted practices like yoga or tai chi to connect with their inner calm. One slim woman I know has been doing twenty minutes of tai chi in her basement, every morning, for more than twenty years. Others find emotional comfort in music. Virtually everyone finds it in nature. Hikers, birders, boaters, and skiers will all tell you that, over and above the particularity of their activity, it is also their direct and personal interaction with nature that powerfully attracts and uplifts them.

"I'm happiest when I'm walking," says one hiking friend who, post-retirement, has made a virtual career of the practice.

One woman I know takes a few moments early every morning to consider an affirmative phrase that sets her up for the day. Another has found tranquility for more than thirty years in Buddhist chants.

I'm convinced that my neighbour who knits experiences an almost Zen-like calm as she settles daily into her well-established routine of knitting beside her front window.

Another friend finds solitary pleasure in needlework. After moving to an entirely new neighbourhood, she also found a new set of friends by starting a needlework group.

For me, it is definitely my early morning walks, my thirty minutes with just myself and the amazing world around me, that give me the quiet and the peace I need.

A recent walk in gentle mist following an overnight rain was an almost religious experience. The flowers, shrubs, trees and even sidewalks of my quiet East York neighbourhood seemed endowed with a special beauty. The dog-walkers, runners, and fellow walkers appeared to exude a certain calm brought out by that cool, damp air.

As for the next generation, several of my mother's grand-daughters still enjoy their quiet moments with a warm mug of tea.

One daughter rarely passes an evening, when her offspring are finally asleep, without a soothing cup of herbal tea cradled in her hands as she relaxes after the day, catching up with her husband, and checking the news on her tablet.

My slim niece, with whom I passed such a pleasant time eating salads in Scotland, is now a talented young potter and businesswoman, and she takes it one step further. Her calming sips of herbal tea are routinely taken from her handmade, pottery mugs in a way that may connect even more intimately to that famous Japanese practice.

My mother would have been shocked to discover that her simple moments with her cups of tea have been as dissected and considered as I've done here. (She would also be surprised to know that I've kept her complete collection of delicate bone china tea cups. Just can't let them go.) As much as my mother valued those moments, relaxed into those moments – and never understood how I couldn't also enjoy a beautiful cup of tea – she would have found it strange indeed that I now view those restful moments of hers as valuable ceremony. But I do.

Of course, the chocolate bar makers of the world would be more than happy if we all chose their products in order to create respite, reward, and calm in our busy lives. But, there are other paths we can take; other sources of respite, reward, and calm we can choose. And these paths can be far lovelier, far more beautiful, and far more supportive of a slim life if we choose them wisely.

Even as Adrianna's struggle with the bread department was unique and particular to her, and absolutely critical to her success in weight control, so too I believe each woman's definition of her own tea ceremony will be unique, particular, and possibly critical to her success in weight control as well.

But, you might now say: that's it? What about exercise? What about a diet plan? What about more *details*?

Well, I might say, all of that is commentary. But, it's interesting commentary. And isn't it always commentary that makes us dig deeper, think harder, and learn better?

So, do read on.

In the next chapter you will learn how all my best efforts seemed to fall apart at midlife – déja vu all over again – and I was almost back to square one in terms of managing my weight.

CHAPTER 6

Becoming Fifty

Suddenly, one day – if we're lucky of course – we all wake up and there we are, we're fifty.

Yikes. How did this happen...we say to ourselves. It all seems so sudden. Of course it's not. But none of us really believe we'll actually grow up – or grow old – until it happens.

And now, suddenly, we're starting to feel different.

A whole raft of physical ailments can hit us, or hit our friends. Some, of course, more serious than others.

Suddenly, we find ourselves thickening around the middle in a way we didn't before. Suddenly, our accustomed pattern of eating isn't keeping the extra pounds away the way it used to. Suddenly, we find that the reading on the scale – which, okay, has been slowly creeping upwards, perhaps just a couple of pounds a year, for quite a while – is now telling us that we're 10 pounds overweight, and heading to 15. Fifteen and heading to 30!!! What's going on? What *exactly* is the matter?

Well, first of all, the changes we experience at this time aren't really sudden at all. Most have been gradually entering our lives since we hit our mid-forties. Some of us may just have been more on top of it than others. And some of us may just have been closing our eyes and hoping these little changes were not a permanent part of who we really were.

But no matter how we lead our lives, very few of us get through these years without a significant change to the body chemistry that has been governing our lives since we became adults. Once I passed the age of fifty, I felt rather like Alice in Wonderland encountering the Red Queen. "Faster, faster," the Red Queen would cry, as Alice ran and ran, losing ground all the time.

My eating habits, entrenched over time, saw me gaining weight steadily, seemingly by magic. My weight control habits, also entrenched over time, no longer seemed to work.

Back in my early twenties, I simply had to cut back sharply on my food intake. Since then, although I might have gained a few pounds here and there, it was never an issue. I'd always lost them again within a few days, generally just by cutting back my food intake. I didn't use any particular diet, just a cutback of the clearly calorie-rich and junk-food items. I'd had three children without gaining any appreciable weight, and I'd internalized the need to eat good, healthy, real food in moderation.

Now at midlife, however, a one-week cutback produced nothing whatsoever on the scales. A two-week cutback could produce a half-pound increase! That outcome stunned me; nothing like gaining weight on a diet to prompt the dreaded give-up mentality. This was it, I decided. I was going to be chubby in my post-fifty years. I couldn't fight it. Nothing was working, and I enjoyed my food. What was I going to do?

But, just as when I was twenty, I hated that feeling of an extra 20 and then an extra 30 pounds around my waist. It didn't feel like me. Back and forth I went. Was I going to give in, or was I going to find a new way through this? Logic told me I could lose that weight. Emotion told me I didn't have what it would take to do it.

That situation continued for five to seven years with my weight gradually increasing all the time. Until, dumb as it sounds, I saw a very simple headline in one of those everyday women's magazines that told me the simple truth. There it was, captioning a small sidebar article: "Older people need fewer calories and more nutrients."

Why hadn't I known that before? Not just the fewer calories bit, but the more nutrients? If there is little room in our lives for junk food in the best of times, there's even less room for it when we're over fifty!

Well, we all find certain truths as we need them, I suppose. And that simple truth helped me a lot. For one thing, I felt relieved that I wasn't imagining things. I wasn't secretly scarfing down much more than I had in the past. The way I'd been living had indeed worked okay for years. But now, I needed less.

Imperfect as they may have been, the eating habits that had maintained me on an even keel for years were now causing me to gain. And also, imperfect as they may have been, my earlier approaches to losing weight no longer resulted in lost pounds and inches, they just maintained the status quo.

Well. This was quite the insight. Perhaps everyone else had known this for years, but I had not. New tactics were clearly required if I was going to lose that annoying blanket around my waist. But step one was a conscious thought process about the situation.

This may seem odd to those who have never needed to cut back on food intake and have never experienced the conflicted feelings associated with that effort. But those who have experienced it, especially those who have had an ongoing pattern of gaining weight and losing weight, will understand that I really did have to give this some thought.

I thoroughly enjoyed food. No question about that. When I considered launching into yet another effort to lose this weight, my dominant emotion was one of anticipated deprivation. As well, now thoroughly affected by my post-fifty experiences, I very strongly anticipated defeat – definitely not success!

I looked around and saw many women my age carrying just as many extra pounds as I was carrying – in fact, many more – and I constantly and consciously said to myself: Why should I worry about this? Why not just accept a bit of chubbiness for the rest of my life?

Was I at all willing to make some kind of extraordinary effort, not knowing if I could really do it, not knowing if it would work, giving up, doing without, experiencing all those negative feelings we associate with losing weight? Hadn't I already cut back and failed to lose weight? Hadn't I already tried this quite a few times in the past eight to ten years?

Jumping on the scales after two weeks of what I considered to be a reducing diet had become an exercise in despair.

I waffled and wavered. I went this way and that. I thought about certain of my eating habits in a way that I'd never quite done before. Then, I just wanted to stop thinking about it, and let everything go. I wanted to just embrace the chubbiness.

However, certain thoughts kept coming back: There is chubbiness now, but how far is that going to go? Will I continue to gain? Was I willing to live with that unpleasant feeling around my middle forever?

Not to over-state the situation, but at some point, amid all that thinking, I did make a conscious decision that I really, truly did *not* want the extra 20-30 pounds I was carrying around – not exactly for vanity – but I hated that bulky feeling. It just didn't feel good. I knew the decision was going to entail some discomfort. But, I decided it was a trade-off that I wanted to make.

I wonder if my mother ever made such a conscious decision.

I don't believe she did. I don't believe she needed to. Although she thickened around the middle as she grew older, to my memory, she never carried the 20-30 extra pounds I found spread all over myself. I think her natural discipline and living habits simply carried her through.

So now here I was, post-fifty, determined to do something, but what exactly would that something be? What could work now that hadn't worked in the past?

At that precise moment I truly didn't know.

But somehow out of that convoluted, back and forth thought process that I'd just engaged in, somehow informed by that *eureka* discovery that I needed fewer calories and more nutrients, and somehow out of my maddening muddle of midlife emotions, a few new tactics came to mind, and I determined to try them.

The very first new and different decision I came to was to not step on the scales for six months.

Not since I was perhaps sixteen or seventeen years old had I gone for any length of time without getting on the scales. As a young woman, I may have even checked them almost daily. Certainly, when I was on my weight-loss cutbacks in earlier years, it would have been every three days or so. I had never in all my adult life avoided the scales for a period of time as long as six months. But, it was crystal clear to me that, if I was going to lose weight at all this time – which I wasn't even sure I could – it was going to be a very, very, very slow process.

My small cutbacks for the past several years had been so discouraging: one week of cutbacks and the scale had not even budged. Two weeks of cutbacks and the scales showed that I seemed to have gained some weight! How does that make you feel? How did that make me feel? Terrible, discouraged, and defeated.

On top of that, my weight loss plan could not and would not be all that drastic. I was way too old for that, and I was looking to increase nutrients after all!

So, for the first time in my life, I decided that if miniscule weight loss and miniscule weight gain were going to wipe out my entire effort of will, then I would remain ignorant of all that for a full six months.

There, I said to myself. Done. Down a bit. Up a bit. I will not know. I will not care. I will just persevere for six months and see what happens.

At the same time, I consciously lowered all my expectations, telling myself religiously that I would be happy with the very smallest of losses.

In retrospect, this was an extremely good move. Far more helpful than I'd ever imagined. I would almost say it was the most important element in this new effort except that everything else was also essential. However, this decision set the stage and was critical in maintaining my motivation and long-term focus.

Then, I had to make decisions about the calories. There was no denying they had to be cut.

First of all, I was not going to turn into an exercise addict at this stage of my life. Never was one, and never would be. So, taking out a gym membership was not going to do the trick for me. Not that I believe it really does the trick for anyone, but more on that later.

Secondly, regarding the relationship between age, calories, and nutrition, the penny had now fully dropped. I realized I had to eat less food now *and for the rest of my life!*

Plus, I needed more nutrients!

In some kind of a new-to-me way, I began to internalize the idea that I could no longer afford to "waste" calories on food that had no helpful nutritional value, or on foods that I didn't really enjoy! This idea was evolving into a view not unlike the idea about possessions: that we should only keep items in our lives that are either useful or beautiful. My new thinking was somewhat similar: only keep in my daily diet items that I truly loved, or truly needed. I began to apply that yardstick consciously and broadly.

And thirdly, I was well old enough to know that drastic and short-run diets are dreadful, unsustainable, and hard on the body and mind. I could not go down that path. So my thoughts were turning instead to a shaving, paring, and trimming approach: little bits of calories reduced here and there.

So, taking all that into account, exactly how was I going to rearrange my eating habits to trim calories, increase nutrients, and not drive myself totally mad?

I began at the beginning, with breakfast. I knew I didn't want to change my breakfast routine too much. I was fond of it. For years, it had been a nice morning brew of coffee plus a bowl of whole grain cereal with toasted bran and whole milk. It had served me well for a good long time, so that part of my day could not be a candidate for radical change. I did, however, decide there was an opportunity for a few, non-radical tweaks.

Taking a closer look at the component parts of my morning bowlful, I decided I could reduce by half the actual cereal I was eating, but leave unreduced the quantity of toasted bran. A smallish cut in calories – you could call it a trim I suppose

— but perhaps not a huge loss in nutrients. I also considered the rather generous spoonful of brown sugar that I'd been regularly putting on top. Calories for sure, and a pleasant taste, but can we really claim many nutrients there? I decided to swap that out with a spoonful of raisins. One of my very first "more nutrients" decisions. Still sweet, actually much more complex and satisfying taste-wise than the brown sugar, but offering a little bit more than empty calories.

Hmmm. Perhaps this exercise could work. Could this exercise work? I didn't know, but I did know that I was soon going through far fewer bags of brown sugar while canisters of raisins were cropping up much more regularly on my shopping lists.

So, that was it for my mornings. Very small changes. But, since my mornings happened, well, every single morning, I told myself that these very small changes must surely add up to something over six months. (You can see the usefulness of that six-month mindset.)

As for my morning coffee, we must all have some kind of indulgence in our lives. Mine is coffee. For years I'd been drinking it with about a teaspoonful of sugar. Just a teaspoonful, but I wondered what it would be like to cut that back. I tried a half a teaspoonful, then a quarter, then nothing. Well, surprise, surprise. I found I far preferred it that way. So, that little teaspoonful of sugar was gone. Just one teaspoonful. But it was one more small shaving of calories that would become permanent in my life.

What about the milk or cream in the coffee? This, I admit, I did not change. I also admit that I didn't use milk. I used half milk and half cream. Now, much later, I do use just milk. But back then, during what I think of as my "midlife, bulky-blanket-around-my-middle effort," I just eliminated the sugar.

So these were the relatively small adjustments to my breakfast routine. Tiny, tiny changes. But ones that I could live with – live with indefinitely as it turned out – and they were at least a little bit helpful.

The next change may have had more impact. I'm pretty sure it did. I decided that I would try to move to an extremely small lunch. Extremely small, virtually invariable, and one that took practically no organizing effort or thought on my part. I decided on a small tub of fruit-bottomed yogurt.

I do not now recall how, when, or where this idea came to me. I know part of my reasoning was that making this change at lunchtime meant I didn't have to upset the breakfast and dinner routines that were working for me. As well, I was taking just a half-hour lunch break at that time, which didn't allow much time for a larger or more leisurely meal as I might have at dinnertime.

As people who know me will attest, I'm a slow eater. If there isn't time to eat something slowly, I'd rather not have it. I suppose that's one natural habit of mine that helps with weight control. Finally, I have to admit that I generally wasn't overly hungry at lunchtime. So, if I was going to make some kind of a larger caloric statement somehow in my life, this was where I could do it.

I'm pretty sure this wouldn't be everyone's choice. And I'm not sure that the good folks at Canada's Food Guide would think such a small meal is a good habit. I don't know that my mother would have thought much of it. Lots of people would prefer a salad, soup, or sandwich at midday. Many people would want, or in fact need, more starch, more protein, or just plain more nourishment than that during their working day.

But many people are younger and more physically active than me. And many people are also not me. The thing is: this suited me. And that was pretty important because every decision, every experiment, every choice I made at that time did have to suit me, as I was post-fifty, and as I was in my daily routines in a fairly sedentary job in communications.

Just as my mother and I differed on the role of tea or coffee in our lives, so too there can be no one-size-fits-all, cookie-cutter approach that will suit all Canadian women when we look to prioritize, organize, and sometimes trim back our food consumption. We have to do what suits us individually and also – very important – what *pleases* us individually.

Around this time I read the book that partly inspired this book: *French Women Don't Get Fat,* by Mireille Guiliano. I loved it, but some things left me cold. For example: leek soup. Reading about it, it sounded lovely, and almost magical, as an entry point into the author's first effort at weight loss. Just for the heck of it, I cooked up a big batch. It did nothing whatsoever for me. I didn't see the point. I didn't enjoy it. And I'm pretty sure I didn't finish it.

Yes, I could see the psychological benefit of starting a weight loss regime with what was virtually a liquid diet/fast for a couple of days, but that particular approach wasn't the thing for me at that time in my life.

I mention this not to in any way criticize that book, which I greatly admire, but simply to stress that we need to make our own individual, personal choices when it comes to weight loss if we wish our efforts to continue and to succeed.

Leek soup was not my choice. Individual tubs of yogurt may not be yours. Each of us as individuals has to look at the overall pattern of our day and say: "Okay. This is what I do. For better or for worse, these are my habits. Where do I pare off the calories? Where and when do I think I can live with this or that cutback on a regular basis? When are the times when I know I eat too much?"

The answers are all very individual.

As for me, I had that same little yogurt lunch day in day out for months. Six months, to be exact! And then, even more.

I found that the bit of sweetness in the yogurt gave me an immediate lift. The fat and protein actually satisfied my hunger very well. It was a top-quality brand, one I already liked. It was not low-fat. It was actually quite high in fat. It was not artificially sweetened. And it was thoroughly enjoyable. I ate it very slowly, savouring the creamy texture and the flavours. Then I went for a short walk before getting back to work.

Something I could have added to this routine, looking back on it now, would have been carrot sticks: easy, delicious, nutritious, low-calorie, and a great source of additional fibre. I often have them now at midday.

In addition to my actual lunch, there was something else I had to address during my working day.

Despite my lifelong interest in healthy eating, I had nevertheless slipped into the habit of turning to some kind of small, junk-food snack as a pick-me-up at certain points during my day: sometimes around 11 in the morning; sometimes around 3 in the afternoon.

It was ridiculous. I didn't even believe in eating junk! But somehow I'd told myself that bits and pieces of it now and then were okay. I was working within a larger department, and many of us there enjoyed snacks, so we'd developed a fairly regular pattern of people bringing in treats, which we then shared: doughnuts from some; assorted potato chips from someone else; homemade cookies, quite delicious; chocolates; salted nuts and more.

I'd also become quite fond of little packages of salty, sesame thingies that were sold in our in-building café.

Let's face it, many of us tend to do this. We all do live in the very real world of high-calorie, low-nutrient snack food. Filled with that big bad trio of salt, sugar, and fat, these items give us a kick when our energy flags, they provide distraction when our focus drops, and they are entertainment – yes, entertainment – when we are just plain bored.

Losing my daytime interludes with those little packages of salty, sesame thingies was a no-brainer. But I'm not saying it was particularly easy.

My energy still flagged. My focus still dropped. And there were times during the day when I still felt just plain bored. I had to live through those moments. I had to get up. Walk around. Go have a chat. Drink some hot water. Stretch. Do something. Do anything. Do nothing. Wait for the urge to pass. Think, consciously, about the fact that six months from now I might not have this weight around my middle. Get through it.

And somehow I did.

Frankly, the new lens through which I was now viewing my calorie consumption helped; these items were absolutely and evidently not worth the calories they contained.

As well, to be honest, the general busyness of work made this daytime effort easier. There were many things to do, many demands on my attention, and any urge I felt to have a pick-me-up did not last all that long. So, I did drop that daytime snacking habit, and I did manage to eliminate those empty calories. And that was pretty well it for my working day.

Then came dinner, and then came the evening. Away from my daytime distractions, this would be a different story.

Dinner in my house had long revolved around some kind of protein, a starch, and lots of vegetables: reasonably nutritious meals that I enjoyed and didn't want to change much. After all, how could I cut back on the very foods that provided those additional nutrients I now understood I required?

So, dinner meals, actually, remained virtually unchanged.

I will say that my serving size at dinner meals was not, and is not, an issue. I am a slow eater naturally, and had not been in the habit of eating very large servings for a great deal of my adult life. So, I did not have to deal with that. Others might have to, and if that is you, take some time to think about it because smaller servings and even smaller plates could be a real help if that's your particular issue.

The one dinnertime change I did make was to more consciously try to avoid fat. For example, if I thought of putting butter on potatoes, I'd put less, or none; if there was a gravy or sauce involved, I'd use less.

But then, there was the evening. Ahhh, the evening.

This is the downfall of many of us who get through our days with busyness interspersed with regular meals, regular foods, and regular quantities that we know we should eat. Evenings, however, are different: laced with associations of down time, indulgent time, socializing time, and also alone time.

Except for those exceptionally busy years when some of us are up to our eyeballs taking care of children, it's also, in our culture, usually a sedentary time spent watching TV, sitting in front of a computer, or reading – often with snacks on the side.

It's a time when some of us eat to compensate for tiredness, or to ward off drowsiness. It's a time when some of us eat out of boredom. It's a time when some of us eat out of simple habit. And, it was for me a time when I did all of that.

My evenings always did – and still do – involve a snack at some time or other. And although my dinner meals did not necessarily involve a dessert, my evenings oftentimes did.

Why, I asked myself one evening (before I started my

six-month odyssey) as I was sitting in my favourite living room chair, knowing that I didn't want that 20 pounds around my waist, knowing that virtually any dessert type of food was loaded with calories, did I still feel such an overwhelming desire for a piece of cherry pie?

Not even homemade cherry pie? Not even the best of the best? Why did I want that extra amount of fat, sugar, and starch? Why did the thought intrude into my mind when I really didn't want it to? Why did I feel as if I needed not just one piece, but two? And, what would really happen if I waited, and waited, and waited through the desire?

I don't know the physiological answer to the why. Undoubtedly, scientists can explain it in bio-chemical terms. But what I did finally realize was that when I didn't go get that particular piece of pie, I experienced something that felt to me like anxiety. I felt bad. I felt uneasy. I. Felt. *Anxious.*

This was another bit of a *eureka* moment for me.

I had never really thought about it in that way before. Never put that word to it. Never waited through a food craving and said to myself: what exactly am I experiencing at this moment in time? Never forced myself to experience that particular "mindfulness" sensation.

Getting the piece – or pieces – of pie and eating them took away that anxiety, I realized. Eating the pie made me feel better. For the moment. But. *Big* but. I didn't like the outcome.

I began to conclude that while, for the most part, my diet had been healthy during my childhood and adult life, I had nevertheless developed some kind of dependence on sweet and fatty items. It seemed my mind was telling me I had to have them – or else! It was as if there was a bit of a minor panic going on in my body that only another piece of pie could calm.

Yikes. It sounded awful put that way. I wanted to shrink from the thought. But I persevered. For the first time ever, I began to acknowledge that my desire for food, when I didn't physiologically require it, was linked to not only all the wonderfully happy emotions and memories we associate with "good food, good times," but also to a far less attractive emotion, that being anxiety.

Up until some point in my life, I could accommodate the extra bits of calories that this type of dependent eating entailed. Not anymore, it seemed, or I would be living with this blanket around my waist forever.

And so I decided, finally, post-fifty, and very quietly, to address this. To *try* to address this – as I truly wondered if I could.

I thought of my mother in her later years. Of her soothing cups of tea. Of her sense of caution in consuming too much. Of her diplomatic refusals.

I don't believe she struggled with any issues of midlife weight gain or food-related anxiety, but certainly she did keep ongoing limits on her food consumption. Somehow, I determined, I must return more consciously and more deliberately to the wisdom of my mother and learn to do the same.

Although I had layers of positive, enjoyable emotions wrapped around the wonderful, non-fattening apples, carrots, and blueberries of my childhood, I also had layers of emotions wrapped around the delicious fruit pies my mother would make, the sugar/fat rush of a really good chocolate bar, and the salty/sour tastes of savoury snacks.

And it was in the evening, when the distractions of the day had quieted, that I truly felt forced into dealing with this – and I decided to face it down.

Sitting in my evening chair, watching TV or reading, I felt the anxiety and I let it build. I did not get up or move. I did not go to get whatever sweet thing was calling out to me. I didn't drink my mother's tea. I couldn't drink my cherished coffee; it would keep me awake at night. So I sipped on a cup of hot water.

And I toughed it out. I waited. And waited. And waited.

And what I discovered was that anxiety doesn't kill. Anxiety does pass. It certainly recurs, again, and again, and again. But it also does pass, again, and again, and again. Brain cells can be retrained. And apparently our complicated body chemistry can be revised. Very gradually, and completely consciously, I disconnected that sense of anxiety from the intake of food. And very gradually, over several months, those feelings diminished and finally disappeared.

It was a completely private, internal effort. I didn't tell anyone what I was doing. Frankly, it would have sounded too weird. But it was as simple, and it was as hard, as that.

Aside from the hot water, the only other items I allowed myself in the evenings were fruit or a small dish of yogurt with a touch of raspberry jam.

Somewhere toward the end of this six-month effort, I spent a brief but lovely week in Paris. And it is odd that in that city of fabulous pastry shops and constant gastronomic delights, I should come to discover another small prop in my trim-down journey.

I was following all my new, more careful habits during that trip. Enjoying immensely the fabulous *café au lait* on offer – no sugar needed. And, pastry lover that I am, wandering in and out of many a *patisserie* during our stay, sampling, with discretion, the odd *pain au chocolat* here, the odd *Madeleine* there, and, *bien sûr*, a slice of *gâteau opèra*. When in Paris, after all.

But, I was pleased that I was not overdoing it. Plus, we were walking everywhere.

It was near the end of our stay that we wandered along the

rue Mouffetard one evening and bumped into a narrow market lane crowded with bottles of wine, displays of fish, many small shops, and the odd restaurant. We wandered up and down, staring, bemused, in our touristy way, at this jumble of offerings. Paris is Paris. There is nothing really comparable in Canada. So, as tourists do, we were busy storing up memories.

We were about to leave, when I noticed, there in the front display of a narrow and unassuming grocery outlet, a type of baked good I had not seen anywhere else during my Paris stay, despite my many diligent pastry shop investigations. I forget the name, unfortunately, but it did have one, hand-written on a little folded card that was propped atop the cake.

This was not one of those elegant, individually shaped pastry items that seem to define so many French desserts. Nor was it an elaboration of cream puff and caramelized sugar. No. It was a rectangular baked cake, golden brown in colour, still in the pan, and cut into squares. No icing. The sign said it contained figs and walnuts. It was sold by the slice. It was not expensive. It was my last day in Paris. I didn't hesitate much in making my decision to purchase.

It was getting late, it was also getting dark, and I didn't actually unwrap or sample this item until much later that evening, after we'd made our pedestrian way back through the Latin Quarter, back across the broad expanse of *les Invalides*, back through the narrow and quieting streets with their occasional views of the city's looming and iconic tower, to our modest hotel.

But when I did taste that cake, perhaps it was end-of-day hunger, perhaps it was an overdose of romantic nostalgia, perhaps I just fell prey to the intoxicating effect travel can have on our senses, but regardless, I thought it was better than any cake or pastry I had eaten in Paris that week. And I'd eaten a few.

It was not extremely sweet. Rather, it was a simple, homey type of cake, moist and quite dense, with the flavours of the figs, walnuts, and spices permeating all and providing an intensity of flavour that was only minimally related to sugar and not at all to chocolate.

Somehow, this was quite an insight for me.

That here, in this city of carefully concocted éclairs, and meringues, and fabulous chocolate everythings, on this sloping, clattering, crowded, narrow, little street, in this unpretentious little grocery shop that offered the usual little bit of this and little bit of that and was most certainly not gourmet in any sense of the word, I would find this delicious little cake that seemed to have come to Paris straight from someone's provincial kitchen, and that was so wonderfully satisfying.

Perhaps only someone with a lifelong love of baked goods can quite comprehend my excitement. I know it sounds a tad over the top, but stumbling onto this item conjoined immediately with my newfound need to make each of my calories count. And I came home from Paris, entered my Canadian kitchen, and promptly started experimenting with spice-infused, mildly sweetened, fig and walnut cakes. And that is how I got onto figs. Calimyrna figs to be exact.

I discovered, by this complete accident, that two or three dried Calimyrna figs, (which, their package will helpfully tell you, deliver a mere 120 calories per three figs) provided a particular type of taste and a particular type of sweet intensity that I enjoyed very much for an after-dinner evening snack. But, they did not, at all, entice me to overdo.

I didn't feel I was "wasting" calories with figs. They were nutritious, after all. I could eat them extremely slowly – nibbling them really – hot water on the side. And, they provided a feel-good, small indulgence that was another reliable prop as I dealt with my evenings.

This accidental Parisian *Mouffetard* encounter, by the way, had another long-term beneficial effect. It got me started on the path of experimenting with fruit and nut cakes in general.

Long the butt of jokes and annual contemptuous assumptions that "no one likes fruitcake," these old-time favourites are still high on the consumption list, year-round, in the United Kingdom. Where, by the way, you can now find absolutely amazing "fat-free" versions in certain high-end cafeterias. Packed with wonderful nuts, I should add, but nevertheless free of the nasty *processed* fats.

At any rate, starting with that street-side, Parisian epiphany – and with little relation to what I know most of us do here in Canada – I've come to think that when you have to balance calories with nutrition, homemade fruitcakes are a great way to have your cake and eat it too. And if you can't routinely stroll into high-end cafeterias in Britain to grab a slice, fruitcakes made at home are definitely the best.

But, to return to my evenings living with anxiety's rising tides: now, in addition to my hot water cure, my small dishes of yogurt and my fruit, I also latched onto figs. And it was relaxing, knowing there was simply never the chance I would overdo on them. Sweetly enough, they also always reminded me of *rue Mouffetard*.

Finally, I will add that during the entire six months I avoided chocolate almost completely, knowing, as I did and as I still do, how difficult it is for me to stop at one small sampling of that particular substance. The short week in Paris was an exception, but even there, most of my food adventures were of the non-chocolate, more savoury variety.

As well, while I avoided all junk food and all desserts, I particularly avoided pies and cashews. That was the Adrianna part of my particular journey.

So, for me, that was about it. The sum total. That was my post-fifty effort to eliminate the bulge.

Six months of avoiding the scale – something I'd had never, ever tried before – six months of very small lunches, cups of hot water, very small cutbacks, swapping foods with empty calories for foods with nutrients, confronting anxiety, avoiding foods that I knew I couldn't control, eliminating junk and all dessert-type items, no additional exercise other than my usual daily walks, the discovery of figs, very small changes and a very slow loss that added up, in the end, to about 12 pounds worth of change on the scale.

!!!!!

I truly couldn't believe it when I gazed down at the scale, six months later, and the needle had finally, finally, finally moved in that downward direction! Not just by two pounds, not just by six pounds, but more than ten. A real difference that I hadn't been able to achieve for seven, eight – maybe even ten years! It was a tremendous breakthrough.

I was so delighted that I just kept on going. The psychological effect of the scale in this case being all positive! I immediately set another scale moratorium of about four months. And it seemed easier, now, as I continued. My new habits were working. It felt great that the blanket around my waist was reduced.

Ultimately, in about the same time frame, I lost 12 more pounds and, in the end, close to 30. The good news is: I've kept it all off.

I no longer routinely have that little, tiny, yogurt lunch, unless I want to, although lunch is always fairly small. If I happen to eat out – and therefore eat more for lunch – I'll rarely eat a large dinner. Fruit and yogurt are still my evening go-to snacks. And I still love my soothing and relaxing cups of hot water.

I have let the occasional dessert and piece of chocolate back into my life; all, of course, in Mum-style moderation.

One important and helpful habit I've kept is the scale moratorium. Except now it's a much shorter timeframe; I weigh myself once a week.

Those who haven't struggled with weight may find this sensitivity/attraction toward news from the scale unnecessary. But those of us who have struggled will know that we always do want to know just where we are. And we're always a bit nervous that we may have gained.

It's not unusual for some of us to feel compelled to check our weight daily. But for me, frequent checking had become too laden with power, too likely to produce feelings of anxiety or defeat, so this once-a-week compromise is my happy medium.

Even so, for several years after my midlife effort, I played a little mental trick on myself before each weigh-in. First, I stood on the scales without lowering my eyes to the reading. Then I told myself I had probably gained. Then I repeated to myself that it did not matter. Then I told myself that I would return to the very small yogurt lunch. Then I told myself that I would be all right. Then, breathing calmly, I would look at the scales.

I confess, more than ten years later, I still sometimes do that when I think my week has been a little over the top. And I further confess that sometimes, when I know I have gone a little over the top, I am still tempted, as I would have done when I was 21, to weigh myself the very next day. I resist. I tell myself Saturday will do. And I wait. This psychological exercise works for me.

People meeting me now assume that I have always been slim. I assumed the same about someone I met quite recently.

But as I told Alya about this book, it quickly emerged that she'd accomplished an even larger drop of 60 pounds, some 30 years ago. Her weight never returned, but we agreed, with a laugh, that whether we remember ourselves as "big," or "large," or "chunky," we never forget how those extra pounds felt. And we're always aware that somehow, some way, those bothersome pounds might come back.

My weight loss wasn't huge or dramatic, I know. I didn't talk about it at all. It happened over an extended period of time, and most family members and friends barely noticed. Some commented later, with a slightly puzzled look, that "You stay very slim, don't you?" Others said that it looked as if I "had lost some weight lately."

But I know and remember how I struggled with those feelings and doubts. The 30 pounds I lost were 30 pounds that really irritated me and really mattered to me. The effort to lose them represented quite a hump for me, and I am truly glad I got past it.

So, thanks Mum. It may have taken awhile for your example to fully sink in. But it finally did.

CHAPTER 7

Being Jamie Salé

The good news about exercise is that moving our bodies is a truly great Canadian pastime.

The bad news is that this doesn't apply to all of us, nor do we apply it all of the time.

Our everyday world is full of distractions – including the time we devote to simply making a living. And many of us find it hard to prioritize exercise.

I'll say this upfront: I do not advocate for exercise as a way to lose or even to maintain our weight. Why? Because it takes a *lot* of exercise to lose a single pound of weight. Most of us just won't do that much. And we're fooling ourselves in a very unhealthy way if we think we can exercise our way to slimness while continuing to overeat.

Pounding away on a treadmill for hours on end just so we can overindulge in food that isn't good for us is simply counter-productive. It's overdoing it in both areas which is never, ever good for our bodies.

I do, however, definitely advocate for moving our bodies regularly, in some form of enjoyable exercise. It is absolutely one of the most important things we can do to maintain a healthy and balanced life physically, emotionally, and mentally.

In Canada, we have one of the best places in the world to do this.

Many a Canadian, small-town backyard is flooded with water and turned into a skating rink for kids every winter across the country. Friendships formed on that Canadian ice frequently continue long into adult life.

In some of Canada's bigger cities, neighbours have been known to remove fencing between adjoining backyards so they could flood a decent-sized space for kids to skate. Certain brand-new housing subdivisions devote more advertising space to small but mighty outdoor skating rinks than the floor plans of their new homes.

Canadians do love their hockey, whether it's the professional teams we follow doggedly, year after year, or the after-work and even post-retirement teams many love to join.

A friend of one of my daughters is one such enthusiast. Slim, trim and energetic, she met her husband-to-be as they battled it out across opposing lines of their respective after-work hockey games. Their eyes locked, he switched teams – sweet, eh? – and the rest became their history as their new and rather more personal team took shape.

Across the country, thousands of girls fill local arenas and twirl across the ice as they dream of being the next Jamie Salé.

Ice sports are unquestionably popular in Canada, but we have so much more to enjoy as well. Not least: fabulous lakes sprinkled generously throughout the country and masses of swimming pools in cities and towns where we can swim easily and cheaply.

An Ottawa cousin loved water sports when he was young and now finds equal pleasure in the hours he spends fishing. But he decided, a few years ago, that his life as a father should include determined efforts to "embrace the winter" with his pre-teen daughters.

Now, this is Ottawa we're talking about. Ottawa, that seems to be directly in the path of all the storm systems that ever blast their way through eastern Canada. Ottawa, that has no problem whatsoever producing a very real Canadian winter with very real Canadian coverings of lots and lots of snow!

Embracing the winter in Ottawa is not a walk in the park.

But weekly winter treks to the beginner ski slopes in the region began. Soon, another family with kids of the same age joined in. It was a determined effort, but it was also fun from the start. And in just a few years, those weekend jaunts produced two teenage daughters who – besides an evident love of fashion – also loved to ski and were likely headed towards a rewarding lifelong habit. Their gift from their father was a true gift to last.

In Canada's gorgeous and mellow Prince Edward Island, residents enjoy long walks on red sand beaches and all kinds of water activities on the rivers and in the cold salt waters surrounding the province during the summer months. But come winter, they're out on their snowshoes – some with their babies in backpacks – tramping its sparkling, snow-covered trails.

Meanwhile, the knockout beauty of Canada's western Rocky Mountains attracts skiers, hikers, and nature lovers of all kinds, all year long. Many of those lucky enough to live nearby leave their cities and towns on the weekend to do what they really live to do: conquer yet another mountain top; ski yet another challenging trail; explore yet another crashing waterfall. Our Rocky Mountains, towering over and straddling both British

Columbia and Alberta, would make anyone an outdoor fan. They're simply magnificent, a tonic to the senses, and a national treasure, full stop.

In my own town of Toronto, the parks and ravines, The Islands (a cluster of islands, mostly set aside as parkland in the city's harbour), the beachfronts on the east and west side of the city, and even a park created out of landfill that juts out into the lake are routinely filled with people running, walking, and biking.

Many Canadians visit the gym, play ultimate frisbee, pursue dance lessons, or play tennis. Many of us run and many play golf. Many take rambunctious dogs for their necessary walks morning and night. Any physical activity that we really enjoy, but especially one experienced in the great outdoors, is one of the greatest gifts we can ever give ourselves.

But, having said all that, it also has to be said, we are not all Jamie Salé.

For those who don't know that name, Jamie Salé is one of our top Olympic champions, a Canadian figure skater *par excellence*, a beautiful and disciplined athlete, a graceful, competitive pro.

Most of us are not like her; what do I mean when I say that? I mean that the trim and toned figures of professional athletes are a wonderful thing to behold. And they do not happen by chance. As much work goes into building and maintaining an athletic body as goes into any other demanding professional endeavour.

We may think athletes have talent. They do. We may think they are lucky. Some are. We may think we should just give up because we'll never be like them. And there's the rub.

Creating an athlete's body is part and parcel of being an athlete. The rest of us, if we want to, can indeed put in that effort. But most of us will not. We should never, however, let that decision or some faulty thought process – *I'll never be as perfect* – stop us from putting in the kind of effort that suits us, that gives us a bit of a lift, and that keeps our body moving in ways we enjoy.

Salé is now a retired athlete and a full-time mum, and she's quick to point out that her focus has shifted away from that hard-driven athletic endeavour. She now works out, as an ordinary person, with a smile on her face, to stay fit, enhance her health, and to enjoy her life and her family.

I admit that I'm one of those non-sporty women who has not taken the time to develop a passion for any organized sport at all. Indoors or out. I'm a very far remove from Jamie Salé. I know it's my loss, but there it is.

For Canadian women like me, fortunately, there is the great Canadian default position, the great Canadian last chance, the great Canadian sport almost *anyone* can do: it's called walking.

Many, many, many Canadian women do this.

Many of us take the opportunity to walk on our lunch hours, fitting it into our normal work routine. Some of us are out first thing in the morning, striding along rural roads, "rails-to-trails" clearances, or city sidewalks. We walk to and from school, in city parks and sheltered ravines. Some women power walk through malls or underground shopping routes during cold Canadian winters or humid summer heat.

It's an activity that's easy, free, requires no special equipment, no special training and can be done anywhere, anytime, for any amount of time. Even when you travel! Maybe, especially when you travel. You can start with five minutes a day and build to thirty. And the nice thing is that your doctor will approve. She'll say, after quizzing you about whether you get any exercise: "Oh, you walk? That's fine. That counts. As long as your heart beats a bit faster and you breathe a bit deeper, that's fine."

Check! Done! I say to myself.

My mother was a walker. A busy, hands-on mum in her younger years, she likely got all the exercise she needed taking care of her little brood. As a working mum later, with much on the go, she would have found it hard to fit any exercise routine into her life. But throughout those years, and then in her later life, she walked. Whenever she got a chance. Even if it was just a quiet stroll in the early evening. As an older woman, she enjoyed it and tried, as much as possible, to get out of the house and walk, virtually every day.

I recently read about a Canadian woman who was living happily, and celebrating a birthday, at the grand old age of 107.

She had experienced heart problems, including angina, some thirty years earlier and had been advised – prescribed, I guess you could say – to walk one hour a day. Clearly a determined individual, she confided, during a newspaper interview, that she'd decided that if one hour was good, she would do two. And apparently she did.

It was all city walking, because that's where she lived. But she was outdoors, moving her legs, breathing the air, just walking: to and fro from her shopping; to and fro from her errands; to and fro from all her regular activities. And she said, that after quite some time, she noticed that her angina had disappeared. Now, here she was, all these many years later, despite those long ago heart issues.

I tell this story not to comment in any comprehensive way on heart disease and angina. I tell it to comment on the ease, the practicality, and the straightforward, well-recognized benefits of walking.

Reflect on that for a moment – ease, practicality, benefits – because now we come to the harder part. While it's great that many Canadian women do exercise in some way or other, what isn't great is that some of us don't, at all. Some of us don't even walk.

In order to turn this around, we need to stop and apply some time, thought and a great dose of self-knowledge to our situations. Even as we forge individual paths when we determine to live slim, we need to make unique and individual choices to avoid being drastically out of shape.

First, let's acknowledge that we don't need to understand in microscopic detail the inner workings of our body to know that exercise is good for us. Our bodies are designed to be busy and on the move. It's that simple. Keeping them active is good for our heart, our lungs, our skin, our lymphatic system, our digestion, our minds: everything.

Knowing this and acting on it, however, are two very different things.

We may have some kind of psychological hump to get over, a sort of looping inner narrative. And it could go something like this: "I know I should, but I can't pump iron or run marathons to lose weight and get in shape. I don't want to pump iron or run marathons. It's boring. I hate exercise. I've never been good at it. It takes too long. I don't have the time. I'll get so sweaty. I won't keep it up. I'll think about this tomorrow. Or next week. Or next year. Tonight, I'm doing TV. TV, with chips."

The first step then is to be thoughtful; to take apart all of our personal thoughts about exercise, take a good look at them, and *disconnect all of them* from having anything to do with weight.

Weight loss and weight control will always – first, last, and foremost – involve controlling our food intake. We have to come to terms with that. The first step will always mean watching that TV with something other than chips on the table beside us.

Next, we have to force ourselves to think of exercise instead as a *treat* to our mental, physical and emotional sense of well-being: a gift; a pleasure; nothing to do with weight at all. And when I use the word force, I am not slipping into over-statement. For those of us who don't naturally gravitate to sports, we really do have to force this.

And finally, we have to think hard about what might work for us. What would we, what could we, enjoy? What can we afford, financially and timewise? Not everyone likes pumping iron or running marathons. Not at all. I certainly don't. Although, I thoroughly respect the thrilling achievements of those who do.

We may have to experiment. Several efforts and trials may not work out. Physical activity is very much linked to generational habits and local opportunities as well as social preferences.

We can think about what our friends are doing. Moving our bodies might be something we want to share with others. It might also be a solitary endeavour we'd really rather do alone. Several of my friends get a great deal of social pleasure from their walking and hiking groups. I tried them, but I have to admit, I prefer the simplicity and quiet of walking on my own.

Moving our bodies can be a night of dancing in one of Montreal's busy nightspots, or an afternoon of line dancing at a local community centre. It can be a game of volleyball on Toronto's summer beaches, or a game of indoor tennis during Winnipeg's long and bitter winter. It can be an early morning jog along the stretching boardwalk waterfront in Charlottetown; or a brisk walk up and down the hilly streets of St. John's, Newfoundland; or an awe-inspiring wander through the cathedral of trees that constitutes Vancouver's Stanley Park.

Moving our bodies can be as simple as a regular walk up and down the flights of stairs in our workplace.

Always it should be enjoyable – not a pain or a duty to avoid.

Here's a key thought that helped me. Some researchers have said that almost all the *psychological* benefits of outdoor exercise happen in the first five minutes of the activity: the lift to the mood; the enjoyment of nature; the simple interaction with others; and the sense that this is truly a grand and wonderful world.

I don't really know if that is true, but I do think there's enough truth in it that we can use the idea as a bit of a stimulant when we find it really hard to get out of the house.

We can trick ourselves into putting on those boots in the winter or getting out the umbrella on a rainy day by saying: "Five minutes, and I'll get almost the entire amount of psychological benefit as if I were out there for thirty."

Of course, once we've walked for five minutes, we'll very likely feel like walking more. Once we've raked the leaves for five minutes we can keep going for twenty. Once we've done a five-minute lap around the pool, we'll want to keep it up.

But I've found, personally, that it's best not to question the trick too much. Better to just let it work. Better to tell yourself determinedly that you're going to go for the five-minute uplift alone, then let the uplift carry you, eventually, to a little bit more.

And on those odd days when you've put in that five-minute effort, and then turn back because, well, five minutes was really and truly all you were good for that day, don't beat yourself up.

Five minutes is always better than none. And there is always tomorrow – as Annie of Broadway fame might say – when the sun will come up, five minutes will become thirty, and some kind of exercise will seem like a lovely thing to do.

CHAPTER 8

A Simple Bowl of Soup

A few years ago, I somehow survived without a kitchen for several weeks as my husband and I took leave of our senses and undertook significant renovations while continuing to live in the house.

A microwave and a toaster oven propped up in the dining room had to suffice, and the array of different ready-made food items we tried was amazing.

Not everything was successful. I'm a home cook, so I find many prepared foods unacceptable for anything but occasional use. But some of our happiest experiences were the soups. I was surprised to discover that many of the mainstream brands had moved well beyond the tinned tomato and chicken noodle standards of my youth. I guess I just hadn't been looking lately.

My mother made soup on a regular basis.

"Waste not, want not" was an understood and often repeated maxim throughout her life. And since we often had roasted chicken as a main meal, we also often had chicken soup which used up all the bits and pieces of that chicken, extracting some of the nutrients from the bones in the process. It was always delicious and is likely the reason I am still so fond of soup today.

But the reason I want to take a little wander into the world of soup is because I believe soups of many kinds can be wonderfully useful props in our efforts to live slim. Consumed during weight loss efforts, the warmth, flavour and high fluid content of a well-made soup can satisfy us both physically and psychologically. They're an excellent way to up our intake of vegetables. Most varieties are healthy, easy to make and delicious. And, leftover soup is a perfect friend in the fridge when we've had too much at lunch and need something simple but lovely for supper.

My mother's technique was utterly simple: simmer the chicken carcass for several hours; remove any obvious gristle and the most awkward bones – she tended to leave in most of the bones and we ate around them; add whatever chopped up vegetables you had in the house, plus rice, salt and pepper, and any other seasonings to taste; keep simmering until everything was done.

There were no measurements; things were done to taste. Her vegetables included carrots, celery, onions, cabbage, turnip, and potato. And it was those vegetables and the remnants of the roasted bird that gave the soup its flavour. She didn't use seasoning cubes. Celery leaves, in particular, enhanced this soup, adding their ever-so-slightly bitter flavour and interesting depth to the broth. My mum never threw out celery leaves, always saving them for the next batch of soup. I still love that distinctive celery flavour.

I had an updated version of chicken soup at the home of one of my daughters recently. She'd made a thin and delicious broth from a recent turkey carcass, poured it over a bed of baby spinach, and served it with large homemade garlic croutons for dunking.

"It's bread soup," she said, as we settled in. Using up leftovers, she'd made something simple, delicious, and satisfying. Her grandmother would have been proud.

The other soup my mother made frequently was a classic beef and barley. Another of my daughters creates her own delicious and wonderful version, full of nutrients, redolent of herbs, and bursting with flavour. Again, her grandmother would have been proud.

I'm a huge fan of pea soups and lentil soups, sometimes seasoned simply with onion, carrots and salt, sometimes seasoned with Indian spices, sometimes seasoned with caraway (try it!).

I don't often make fish soup, but the possibilities there are endless. From *bouillabaisse*-inspired mixtures featuring tomatoes, herbs, and olive oil, to mussels steamed to perfection alongside slivered vegetables in a well-seasoned wine broth, to chowders of all types.

Speaking of chowders: Nova Scotia not only puts its apples on a pretty high pedestal with an Apple Blossom Festival each spring, it also elevates chowder with a "chowder trail" each summer for tourists and residents alike. All over the province, restaurants compete with each other – and with the idea of chowder excellence – to see how close they can get to perfection. There's many a delicious variation, and I have sampled a few.

One of my favourites was one I enjoyed at a flourishing winery, set midway up the rising slopes of South Mountain, in the completely gorgeous Gaspereau Valley. This small river valley is part and parcel of the much larger Annapolis Valley, but has its own distinctive appearance and charm.

This particular winery – one of several in the region – looks down, over, and around to nearby fields, farmhouses, trees and stretching orchards. But its ultimate vista is an outstanding view of the region's extensive tidal river basin which stretches outward in overlapping and almost undulating shades of blue and green and brown and glittering silver: endless beauty all around that reaches and includes the distinctive silhouette of Mount Blomidon, off in the distance.

It's a stunning location, and it's a view that everyone in the area adores.

"It was a rundown old farm when I bought it," said the owner, who happened to be on hand the day I visited.

Now, busloads of city dwellers join locals to enjoy the view, sample the wine, visit a few more wineries while they're at it, and, as I did, linger over a simply lovely meal – including chowder – in the open air.

Quebec has long been famous for its hearty and satisfying pea soup: yellow whole or split peas cooked to a mushy perfection with onion and ham hock completing the picture. It's one of my absolute favourites.

Meanwhile, in the depths of a Charlottetown winter – generally pretty cold, pretty snowy, but pretty darn festive during Christmas week – some of my family members stumbled, one year, on a tomato, fish, rice chowder recipe for their Christmas Eve meal. Simple, warming, satisfying, and tasting all the better the longer it would sit through the evening, it became, through the years, their Christmas Eve tradition. So much so that when one of the younger family members found herself spending Christmas week in France during her student years, this chowder is exactly what she found herself making as Christmas Eve approached, all so she could experience that special feeling of home.

Then, who could forget Thai soups? These I would not try to duplicate at home – some would, I can't – but I absolutely love these soups with their little floating mushrooms, their tastes of lemongrass and coconut, and the warm heat of the various peppers providing their kick.

Minestrone is another personal favourite. While I may not be completely authentic in all my preparations, it isn't hard to find a way to mix red or white kidney beans with chopped vegetables, tomatoes, a bit of good olive oil, some kind of pasta, your favourite herbs and seasonings and simmer it all to a wonderful conclusion. This, too, ages well and tastes even better the following day.

I enjoyed many a delicious and nutritious soup at my mother's table. I've enjoyed many at my own table as well. And as a change from larger, more elaborate and perhaps higher calorie meals, they're an easy, useful and also cost-effective option.

But I've also observed that, as a lovely side benefit, there is something about these fragrant, steaming bowls of soup that makes us want to slow down, as my mother did with her steaming cups of tea, and savour the flavour as well as the positive value of what we are eating.

And when we're shifting habits of over-consumption to habits of moderation, this slowed-down focus on nourishing food, consumed quietly and with appreciation, can only be a good thing.

CHAPTER 9

What to do about Sweets

Okay, so we all have a fondness for sweets.

Well, perhaps not absolutely everyone. I do have one daughter who would rather eat an olive any day over something sweet. And she has a knack for turning everything under the sun into the most amazing salads: pumpkin seeds; artichoke hearts; radicchio; goat cheese; napa cabbage; toasted walnuts; shaved fennel; spiced olives; pomegranate seeds; softened currants; slivered almonds; sliced pear; baby spinach; chopped kale; balsamic reduction; julienned everything. You name it, she's tried it. And her husband appreciates.

But most of us enjoy the taste and – let's be honest – the kick of something sweet.

It's natural that we feel this way. The first thing we taste as we begin our lives is the sweet, fatty liquid that is early breast milk. We may never again find sweetness mixed with fat in as perfect a combination. But we've all become adept at creating sweet/fat combinations that please our palates well beyond those baby days.

Plus, as far as we know, our species has long evolved on the taste of sweet. Fruits, berries, seeds, nuts, vegetables, milks, grains, and legumes all contain some kind of sugar or starch that registers on our palates and brains, telling us that this food is good.

And, the fact is, this is true. Our brain knows that we do indeed need natural sugars and starches to function.

But the problem is that our brains and our palates are intensely malleable and easily led astray, in all kinds of ways. While this malleability is a part of everything that is alive, an essential attribute that ensures life's ability to adapt and survive, it can also have a significant downside.

All sugars and starches – including worthwhile ones contained in worthwhile foods – provide an immediate lift to our blood sugar levels and our moods. They taste good, they make us feel good, and our neural network responds appropriately, telling us to seek them out. All too easily, this message permeates our being: "*Anything* sweet is good. Eat more!"

This wasn't a bad thing in times when much of the sweetness we enjoyed came from natural and often-scarce foods like berries, whole grains, fresh or dried fruits, and yes, even milk. Foods we had to work hard to acquire, work hard to make edible or palatable, and work hard to preserve for the times they were out of season.

But mass-produced foods of all kinds – and especially mass-produced sugars – long ago changed all that. Our poor, bewildered brains now have a very tough time distinguishing between what seems good and what really is good.

Living slim and healthy can no longer be left to our impressionable neural network that insistently sings: "Anything sweet is good."

That works just fine during our first year of life when breast milk is indeed sweet and good, changing naturally and as needed from that first, concentrated mixture of sweet and fatty nutrition to the thinner, but still slightly sweet mixture that provides every bit of the protein, sugar, fat and nutrients – as well as tons of fluid – that we need.

The minute we move on from that, however, we can very easily get into trouble. Just watch any toddler being given his or her first sampling of birthday cake – with icing! We all know the reaction there. Generally a fair bit different from their first sampling of cooked zucchini.

From that moment on, we must consciously sing to ourselves: "Sweet is not always good. Sweet must be sampled in moderation. Sweet will control us if we don't actively control it."

Well, of course, yikes!

That's a bit of a heavy message for any toddler. And it's a bit of a heavy message when it's such seemingly wonderful, delightful food concoctions we may be talking about, and when so many of these seemingly wonderful, delightful food concoctions are at the core of beloved family celebrations and cultural traditions.

I haven't forgotten the absolute pleasure I took in the many family birthday cakes of my childhood. I haven't forgotten the very first time I tasted a particular brand of purchased cookie that included a cookie base, marshmallow filling, and chocolate covering. I was at a kid's birthday party, and I thought I was in heaven.

I haven't forgotten how, as a teenager, I worked to perfect the art of homemade icings so they were perfectly creamy, perfectly smooth, and perfectly perfect. I carried this on to the celebrations of my own children's happy birthdays as well.

But sugar is a dangerous friend and, as adults, we ignore this at our peril.

Ours is now a world where each and every major holiday has sweet and fundamentally unhealthy items specially created, branded, and marketed to celebrate the occasion. Ours is a world where even the sound of the little metal top snapping off a fresh can of cold pop can fill some people with a rush of anticipatory pleasure. This is not the world of special-occasion-only, home-made treats into which my mother was born.

Naturally, no child stepping up to this imperfect smorgasbord of adult food begins any habit of sugar restraint on his or her own. Parents and caregivers do it for them. We ration Halloween candies. We encourage real food first, desserts a distant and only occasional second. We understand about "sugar highs." And we know that pop is a nasty, sneaky monster that lurks everywhere in a child's life.

But, it's a tough sell. And it continues to be a tough sell for the long haul, living, as we do, in a time, and a culture, and a place, where sugars are everywhere.

In this respect, Canadian women face the same challenges felt by everyone touched by mass food production. Over and above overtly sweet items, sugars permeate our prepared foods to kick up flavour, to preserve them, and even to create textures we find agreeable.

This isn't going away anytime soon. So, how do we navigate through this sugar-filled world and remain slim and healthy in spite of these pressures?

Once again, we must battle neurons with neurons, imagination with imagination, value system with value system, and enjoyment with enjoyment.

Once again, we must look critically at commercial food

enterprises and turn away from the sugar-filled concoctions they've churned out, in mindless lockstep, over the last many years. We must challenge fake food with real food, embracing a livelier and more interesting world of sweet built around the flavours of real, natural foods that satisfy us fully, mind, body and soul.

One of my most delightful sweet memories is of a real sugar shack, in the winter, in rural New Brunswick. It's a great memory. Pristine. Locked in my memory and magical.

As with so many great food memories, it's linked to family and beautifully placed in the great outdoors.

We lived, at the time, for one full year only, on a country road not far from Salisbury, New Brunswick. It was my one and only experience of attending a one-room schoolhouse, and I loved it.

That winter, snow lay deep and delightful all around our small home, stretching over the farmlands that surrounded us and resting soft and fairy-like on the trees and shrubs that lined a nearby brook. I enjoyed that brook. The way it meandered, broke into two streams, circled around a tiny "island" and then continued on its way. I played near it in the warmer seasons, living out adventures created by my childhood imagination. But, I'd never ventured up its farthest reaches – that was a place of mystery – until winter reached its turning point and maple syrup time commenced.

Sugaring-off was a time-honoured local tradition, as we soon discovered.

In my father's family of Nova Scotian farmers, small-scale sap collection and the making of syrup had been a longtime custom. But for us youngsters, this was our first – and only – winter on that rural New Brunswick road, and this particular evening excursion was entirely new. We tramped back together, all five of us, my mother, my father, my brother, my sister and I, following the brook's course, back to that small wooden shack nestled amidst the trees. Huge billows of steam emanated from the building. Inside, giant vats of maple sap were evaporating their way towards maple syrup over the glowing fires.

That night shines in my memory. Perhaps it was a slightly spooky adventure for me: setting forth, en famille, into the unknown along the edges of that unexplored brook, only to arrive in a place of warmth and joviality with much of the larger community already there and in festive mode.

We kids watched and learned. And eventually, we were given our own ladles of hot syrup to take out of the shack, to pour directly onto some fresh clean snow, and then to taste. I doubt that maple syrup has ever tasted as good to me since as it did that night, sampled straight, hardened by the crisp snow, in the woods, under the hard and glittering stars.

After I'd written these words, I wondered if my younger brother and older sister remembered that night as well. "Oh yes," they both said, to my surprise. That memory having lodged so firmly and personally in my own mind, I hadn't stopped to think if it had lodged in theirs.

"That's why I buy a can of New Brunswick maple syrup every year," said my sister. "I keep it in the fridge. I have one there now."

Years later, as I drove with my own family of youngsters through New Brunswick, time and again, on our way to Nova Scotia from Ontario, we'd aim for a quick stop in Sussex for ice cream. It always seemed to taste better in those rural surrounds than anywhere else in the world.

Coffee milkshakes, strawberry ice cream, mocha mixtures — we'd each choose our favourite and, back in the car, savour them slowly as we continued through the flat and spreading beauty of the countryside. That peaceful, slow-moving Saint John River, in the warm summer heat, offered the most gorgeous view you could imagine.

I now have the benefit of a friendly little pink and white striped ice cream shop on a side street just off the Danforth near my home in east-end Toronto. I love to see the kids making their chalk drawings on the sidewalk in front of the shop on a warm summer night while their parents linger and chat.

In Prince Edward Island, another friendly little yellow and white striped ice cream shop offers quite a contrast.

Set in a charmingly updated older home and just opened by my niece, it delivers views of broad, sweeping patchwork fields: a vista of gently sloping green, gold and brown. The delightful draw of its sweet offerings sees kids and their parents, and others too, linger and chat, hop on a hammock, or run around on the grass.

Sweet things have a definite place in our lives. They're fun. They belong. We love them. Whether it's the dense, sweet experience of a single, perfect banana, the complex subtlety of a well-made fruit cake, the utter perfection of a lovely orange, or the satisfaction of a warm and delicious blueberry pie, Canadian women – and men for that matter – aren't about to follow any eating regime that means no such sweetness in their lives.

"Oh, I love date squares," said the sturdy, blunt-spoken Nova Scotia farmer, whom I met, one day, when he was visiting his friend, my elderly uncle, in the hospital.

The topic was health, and the conversation was circling around diabetes, because my uncle's friend, who was in his late '50s, lived with the condition and was managing quite well, thank you very much. But, did he ever eat sweets?

"Oh, I won't give up a good date square," he said. "They're

my favourite. I'll have a date square, now and then. Oh, for sure. But, it's just now and then. Not every day. And what I'll do is this: I'll just watch anything else I eat that day. And, I'll get in some more exercise. Even if I go out and walk down the lane for 20 minutes or so, it brings my blood sugar right down. Right down. Oh no, I can still eat a good date square."

Fortunately, most of us don't need to exercise quite the degree of caution required of someone living with diabetes. And full respect here, also, for those who have to be more cautious for any reason of health.

But all of us do need to exercise caution, and to come to terms, in a realistic way, with the world of sweet.

Although it sounds boringly simple, it can be achingly difficult: we must not only bring discipline but also intelligence to bear on this matter. But, our species has been known to put people on the moon, after all. We can figure this out.

Most Canadian mothers, including my own, teach their children the simple lesson that sweet things must be consumed in moderation, as additions to a regular, healthy diet. Not for breakfast. Not before meals. And not ever as routine substitutes for real nourishment.

As adults, we can continue to know this and to understand it in more specific and personal detail.

For example, we can acknowledge that a sweet date, apricot, or raisin carries into our lives exquisite taste as well as the benefits of actual nutrition, but any kind of pop brings only empty calories and the prospect of diabetes. We can understand that a bowl of fresh pineapple or juicy, ripe cherries is a treat that tastes delicious and builds our health whereas too many chocolate chip cookies can damage our health and shorten our lives.

We are only fooling ourselves if we pretend it's not true. We need to make conscious choices about the type, quantity, and quality of sweet items we will have in our lives, even as we learn to choose, with discretion, which friends, jobs, and activities we'll retain as keepers.

Since our nation is one of magnificent cultural diversity, we are magnificently diverse in this area as well.

Those Canadian women whose cultural background dictates Persian cookies for New Year can feel lucky Iran has a longstanding tradition of using apricots, dates, figs, and pistachios in such delicious concoctions. But they can also consider ways to reduce the sugar in any homemade creations and apply moderation as they enjoy these treats with family and friends.

Those Canadian women whose cultural background dictates Caribbean fruit cake at Christmas can feel lucky that their culture has perfected the art of that flavourful combination. But, they can also consider ways to reduce the sugar in their grandmother's recipe and do something about the extremely sweet drinks that may also appear on their festive dining tables.

Those Canadian women of any cultural background who have grown up thinking cookie possibilities start and end with chocolate chips while cakes start and end with a boxed mix, have an almost infinite scope for change.

Nuts and dried or fresh fruits are the classic and still completely worthwhile bases for traditional and delicious sweet treats. They remain the very best places to start. Cookbooks abound while the internet overflows with suggestions. A quick search online for "date bread" can produce some 143,000 results – in less than a second!

It's worth the effort to experiment.

One of my daughters, who is just starting to create her own cookie recipes for her young family, has found that as a rule of thumb she can almost always use about one-third of the sugar called for in any cookie recipe.

Yes, the cookies are considerably less sweet. But yes, they are still sweet enough. And whatever dried fruit or nut is added to the mixture brings its own much more complex and satisfying flavour to the end result as well.

Personally, I count myself among the cookie, bread, and pastry lovers of this world. Perhaps, it was because my mother was a baker and an excellent one at that. Quick and efficient – as I am now too – she turned out crisp yet tender tea biscuits that were delicious topped with jam. She was perfect at pastry. And her favourite hermit cookie recipe became my favourite as well.

Some people are surprised to learn how much I enjoy and appreciate certain baked goods.

"But, you're so slim," more than one person has said to me when I've shared photos or told stories of an unusual baked good that I've tried. As if enjoying a Black Forest cake *in* the Black Forest (a person has to do that, right?) or a bitter orange cake in Australia cannot co-exist with slimness.

Yes, I do love certain sweet baked things, and I enjoy discovering new tastes as I travel or visit with friends, but I eat them only occasionally, they are mostly homemade, and they *must be good enough* to be worth the consumption.

In fact, since my midlife experience, my eating expectations have been so firmly adjusted that my own homemade and wholegrain tea biscuits, sweetened only with currants, slivered apricots and pecans, are incredibly more satisfying to me than virtually any other sweet treat. Yup. Believe it.

And if I do make an occasional moist and fruity gingerbread, or the carrot cake my grandson now expects for his birthday, I don't layer on icing and I don't consider such items to be junk food, the way I categorize chips, candy and pop. Rather, I see them as part of my cultural past and present, a reflection of my personal interest in food, and a rewarding creative endeavour.

So: blueberries, anyone? *With* a drizzle of our beloved Canadian maple syrup? *With* a small topping of the best vanilla ice cream you can find? I say, go ahead. Gild that luscious lily once in a while!

I think my mother felt the same way. In fact, I'm sure she did.

CHAPTER 10

Counting up the Calories

Ahhh, calories.

Once, very much in fashion. Once, very much considered when thoughts or discussions turned to diets. Once, more or less elevated to an all-important, high priestess status if you were dealing with too much weight – or too little weight.

Now, calories are the forgotten and sometimes-disparaged former best friend.

Well, I'm going to talk about calories. Because they are a fact of life, and I think it's helpful to understand them.

But notice where they come in the book. Not exactly at the beginning, eh?

And if you really can't bear to read about them, go ahead and skip this chapter, or take a short-cut, because to reduce calories without calculations, you can always just reduce portions. It can be as simple as that.

But I am going to be un-simple and probe a bit more.

What exactly are calories?

Calories are a measure of the amount of energy stored in foods that becomes available to run our bodies once we consume and digest those foods.

Calories are a measurement of energy in the same way pounds and kilograms measure weight and pints and litres measure volume.

Speaking in very general terms, if you're a woman who weighs about 110 pounds, you need, on average, 1860 calories to keep you going each day, to run your body with all its component parts, without gaining or losing weight.

If you weigh 120 pounds, you'll need about 1950 calories. If you weigh 165 pounds, you'll need about 2400 calories.

It's worth taking a bit of time to think about that. You can see straightaway that the heavier you are, the more calories it takes to run your body.

While we can dance all we like around varied dieting advice – from grapefruits, to blood types, to ancestral habits, to Mediterranean customs – there's some basic math involved in eating just enough food, containing just enough calories, to keep us both slim *and* healthy.

It's not unlike the math involved in pouring ten ounces of water into an eight-ounce cup. That cup will hold eight ounces no matter how much you hope, wish, or dream that it will hold more. The rest of the water, those extra two ounces, overflows.

We do ourselves no favours to ignore this.

One interesting aspect to this calorie math: *most* of the basic number of calories we need on a regular basis every day – the numbers noted just above – are used *simply to maintain the regular internal functioning of our body itself.*

It seems amazing, but it's true.

Many of us have internalized a belief that our bodies are

only using up energy when we're out on an early morning jog, working up a lather at the gym, or racing around the house chasing babies and kids.

That's simply not the case.

If we lie on the couch all day and do nothing energetic whatsoever, our bodies still need a basic number of calories to keep going. Less than if we were busy, it's true. But still quite a sizeable chunk.

We still need energy (calories) to keep our hearts ticking, our brains cleared of dead cells, and our digestive systems functioning. We need energy to produce new blood cells, grow new hair, keep tear ducts operational, create new fingernails, produce multiple hormones, and to keep bones and bone marrow cleared of waste.

Even to dream takes energy! Our brains are very busy taking care of themselves while we sleep.

I sometimes think of our bodies as busy factories of creation and destruction, because that's exactly what they do: create and destroy; build up, tear down; manufacture something incredible, use it, then clean away the mess, all day, every day, every day of our lives.

And all of this happens, for the most part, below the radar of our conscious observation.

Oh, we can certainly notice our body's busy efforts when we fall sick and our immune system goes into overdrive getting rid of a virus. We feel those effects: all that coughing; all that sneezing; all that awfulness.

But when we're well we rarely acknowledge, think about, or say thank you to our kidneys, our pancreas, our lungs, our inner ears – all the bits and pieces that keep working quietly, day in day out, while our conscious selves get to admire sunsets, go to movies, and enjoy our lives.

But every single bit of this takes energy. Whether or not we ever lift weights or dive into a pool. Whether or not we ever leave that couch.

Take the example of a woman who weighs 165 pounds.

She may be the very same height as the woman who weighs 120 pounds. But, because her body is bigger and heavier, she needs more calories to maintain her body. She simply has more cells to nourish, more blood to replenish, more skin surface to clean and replace, more everything. Her heart also has to work that much harder to send more blood into more places. That's why she needs 2400 calories to maintain her weight while her 120 pound sister only needs 1950.

If our 165-pound friend dropped her intake of calories to 1950, she would be consuming fewer calories than she needs to supply her daily energy needs. Her body would not stop producing hair or fingernails. It would not stop manufacturing and creating, destroying and cleaning. She would not stop breathing, or sleeping, or dreaming.

But, because she's consuming less energy than she needs for all of this, her body would now turn to some little bundles of stored energy it had produced and set aside earlier on. Because, unlike the extra water that spilled out of the eight ounce cup when we tried to fill it with ten ounces, the extra calories that go into our bodies are not spilled out. Rather, they are saved, made into fat cells, and stored carefully away in different parts of our bodies, just in case.

Our bodies do not throw away the superfluous energy that comes their way, *just in case* they need that energy later.

Our human bodies are the ultimate hoarding machines. During our long evolution, we have known feast and we have known a great deal of famine. And like all living organisms, we have survived by developing ways to get through both.

Our bodies exist in a continual flurry of possibility. And, as does any creative enterprise when faced with a challenge, our bodies try their best to develop a solution, or at the very least, a work-around. Their solution or work-around in this particular situation has been to create many new little cups called fat cells. Our bodies create them, fill them with the overflow calories, and then store them in preparation for times of famine.

The body of our 165-pound friend will now turn to those little stored cups and it will change them into the energy it needs to do all its daily chores. As these little collections of fat are used up, our friend will experience a gradual drop in her weight until she reaches 120 pounds.

At this point, she will be eating the amount she needs to provide the energy to maintain her body. At this point, her body, in its wisdom, will stop seeking out and using its fat cells. So, at this point, she will stop losing weight.

Knowing this helps us understand why we get discouraged at certain points during a weight loss regime.

Let's just say our friend really wanted to reach a goal weight of 110 pounds. If she was consistently consuming 1950 calories, she would gradually drop in weight to 120 and then, even though she had not changed a thing in her eating regime, she would stop losing. She may think: it's worked so far; why has it stopped working?

At this point, if she really does want to lose more, she'll have to reduce her calorie consumption even further to continue losing weight.

The fact that we need more calories to maintain heavier bodies also helps us understand why so many of us get caught in yoyo diets.

We may have been consuming those 2400 calories, or more, for quite some time, and we may have been really enjoying the food habits we'd thereby developed.

When we finally reach 120 pounds, we think: great, now I can *really* eat again!

And back we go to our pattern of 2400 calories. Perhaps more. Because we've been missing some of those foods quite a bit.

Big mistake.

Our 120-pound body does not need that amount. Never has. Never will. We're right back to the situation of the over-flowing cup.

Our famine-conscious bodies will now start to sock away the extra, bit by bit, day by day, usually back into the very same cells we have just emptied of fat, until we're right back up to the level where we were before. At that point, if we continue to consume 2400 calories, we will level off in weight gain at the 165-pound mark because our larger body again needs that larger amount of energy to maintain itself. If we consume even more, we'll just continue to gain.

The bottom line is this: if we have made an effort to slim down – and have actually succeeded – we have to come to terms with that fact that our newly slimmer bodies now need fewer calories – now and forever – to maintain their normal, essential, internal functions.

This is a fact. Better we know it and deal with it than to stubbornly try to fool ourselves and swing up and swing down in a never-ending series of gains and losses.

But, let's go back to the couch with all that busy activity going on inside us while we lie there, dreaming of our next vacation.

Well, of course, we don't do that day in, day out.

Naturally, we leave that couch. We do all kinds of great and wonderful things. And our kidneys and pancreas keep ticking away, even as we go to work, go to school, take care of the kids, visit the gym, run our errands, visit great-aunt Monica, and do whatever.

But *most* of the calories and energy that *most* of us consume each day goes to maintain this internal, everyday functioning of the body. Only a smaller, additional portion is needed to ensure we get to work and school, take care of the kids, visit the gym, run our errands, and visit great-aunt Monica.

Looking to physical exercise for a weight-loss benefit can be a way of avoiding this basic fact. Yes, we can burn up a bit more energy by exercising, but we'd have to do an awful lot of it to result in weight loss.

Professional athletes and even some amateur sports enthusiasts may burn through mega-energy and mega-calories in their exercise routines. But they also see their appetites increase enormously – along with their nutritional needs – and that is a whole other consideration.

Most of us simply will not exercise enough to lose significant weight. Most of us can't and won't spend hours at the skating arena or in the swimming pool each day. Most of us can, however, exercise moderately simply for the pure joy of it and the many outstanding health benefits it provides.

On average, people need to consume about 3,500 extra calories – that is, 3,500 more than you need to run your body and do your normal activities – to add one pound of fat to their bodies.

Correspondingly, most people who reduce their calorie intake by the same amount will lose about a pound of body fat.

So, consuming an extra 500 calories a day, over just one week, normally adds about a pound to your weight. And, a reduction of 500 calories a day, for just one week, normally sees you drop about a pound.

Calorie counting was not an activity my mother wanted, or needed, to care much about.

Her deeply held eating rituals and patterns kept her far away from junk food for the most part and she enjoyed good, fresh food far too much to be knocked off her well-worn path by the commercial food industry. Healthy eating was a culturally entrenched value for her and one she delivered emphatically to her children.

She didn't need to study a calorie booklet to know that a small piece of dessert was all she needed or wanted, or that chocolate was a small treat to be enjoyed just once in a while. Her quiet pragmatism and innate appreciation for order meant she was naturally disinclined to overindulge.

But, growing up, myself, in the '50s and '60s, I did study calorie-counting booklets – intently – so I was aware of the approximate energy value of most foods.

Not as fortunate as my slender mother in terms of natural self-control, I also chose to ignore this information frequently when it came to chocolates, chips and baked goods.

As North America's obesity epidemic worsened during the past century, diet approaches changed along with it. A simple focus on calories became less fashionable, replaced with specialized, heavily branded approaches complete with books, spokespeople, and – sometimes – specially prepared foods.

It's strange when you think about it: the commercial food industry playing such a huge and profitable role *creating* obesity; the commercial food industry playing such a huge and profitable role *fighting* obesity.

You've heard the expression? They get you coming and going.

Calorie counting alone is certainly not enough to anchor our efforts when managing our weight. While the raw numbers might appear the same, there is no health equivalency between the calories contained in a mellow and marvelous avocado and the calories contained in store-bought cake listing sugar as its first ingredient.

But knowledge is power, or, at the very least, strength. So knowing the approximate caloric content of basic foods and the approximate caloric level you need to maintain your body is, in my view, helpful if you've had any difficulty at all with weight.

Calorie counting booklets can still be found in some stores, but the information is also now broadly available online, as are sites or apps that tell you how many calories are required to perform various types of activities or exercise.

As one young adult in my life said when he realized just how much additional time he'd have to expend on a treadmill to equal the calories consumed in just one cookie: "It made a whole lot more sense just to forego the cookie."

A bit of time devoted to figuring it all out is extremely worthwhile and, in my view, solidly helpful to any Canadian woman interested in living slim.

CHAPTER 11

Amélie's Story: The Lonely Carrot

I was seated at a round, white-tablecloth-draped table as I made my delicious way through a wedding dinner in an enormous, red-brick, converted armoury. The location: a small, south-western, Ontario farming town.

The bride's family lived here, not far from the protected reaches of Point Pelee National Park. A favoured stopover location for migratory birds and butterflies, Point Pelee extends deep into Lake Erie, the Great Lake that, in this part of Canada, is the effective border between our country and the United States to the south.

Spreading in unending flatness around the town, beyond its concentrated grid of tree-lined streets and gracious homes, were the wide, hazy fields of a verdant countryside: the late summer green of corn, potatoes and tomatoes.

City-dweller that I've become, I was only able to recognize the corn. Despite a dry summer, a seemingly lush set of crops shimmered all around us under the high, blue sky.

We had made it an excursion, my husband and I, coming from Toronto and staying overnight, so we could explore the town and the area.

It was now early evening of the wedding day and, on the table in front of me, the wedding feast unfolded. It began with a tangy red pepper bisque followed by delicate garden greens dressed with a gentle raspberry "pull." The main event: a choice of outstandingly tender steak or sea bass served with grilled asparagus, mashed potatoes, and a large, delicious steamed carrot, rustic in its cut and simple presentation. Comfort food, and traditional hearty Canadian food, beautifully prepared.

It was a meal that seemed to celebrate the farming traditions we had witnessed all around us that day. Traditions, I mused, that had likely been part of the bride's entire life.

It was also a meal that my mother would have found pleasingly familiar: a presentation that was about two-thirds fresh vegetables and 100 percent real food.

Yes, it was fairly hearty, to be sure. And it was probably more than my sixty-something body would have ideally wanted or consumed at home. Thankfully, the crème caramel was a light touch at the end. But the measured pace of the presentation meant I did indeed make my way through every single bit of it. It was a wonderful, pleasurable, and delightfully homey experience.

Seated next to me was Amélie, a close friend of the mother of the groom. We had that friendship in common. I had known the mother of the groom since our respective children were very young. My tablemate had known her even longer. A charming, upbeat woman, she was, I discovered, exactly my age.

Petite, trim, and stylishly put together, she chatted easily, her speech retaining the gentle shading of the Montreal French of her origins. We talked about children, jobs, grandchildren and weather. Everything and nothing. The usual.

As the courses followed, one after another, from soup, to salad, to plated meal, she was aglow with appreciation for the splendid offerings. She relished the soup, commented enthusiastically on the freshness of the salad ingredients, and was delighted with the steak. Everything on her plate was consumed with enjoyment – except for the large length of that one whole carrot.

As we all finished up – she, my husband, and I – we shared a moment of unanimous appreciation for the perfectly delectable meal.

Then my husband noticed the carrot still lying in lonely splendour on her plate. It surprised him, especially considering her several comments on the quality of the vegetables throughout.

"You've missed something great in leaving that carrot," he couldn't help but say. He can, at times, be just a touch more forthright than me. "They were fantastic."

"Oh, I know," she said quickly. "But, I have to be careful about eating some things like that. I have a medical condition that means I have to be careful about foods with starches and sugars – certain types of starches and sugars – and also salt. I ate the potatoes. I didn't eat the bread. The carrot has a lot of sugar, so I thought I'd better not eat that."

"Oh, are you diabetic?" I promptly asked. Just as promptly, I felt that I had probably asked too personal a question.

"No, I'm not diabetic," she said. "But something similar. I do produce insulin, but my body doesn't use it well. I have something called metabolic syndrome. It's very complicated," she added, with a bit of a gentle smile, as I looked at her somewhat blankly.

I told her I had heard the term, generally connected in some way to information about diabetes, but I really had no idea what it was.

"Well, it's complicated," she said again. "I was sick. Very sick. I couldn't digest my food, and it was very painful. I was diagnosed two years ago and put on a special diet by my doctor. All OHIP covered," she added quickly, using our local short-form for our famously valuable, publicly funded health insurance (Ontario Health Insurance Plan).

Of course, what she really meant by saying this – and what I well understood that it was really code for – was that this was a doctor-supported, mainstream medical treatment, not some weird, off-beat adventure.

She then listed a quick but quite detailed series of dietetic do's and don'ts that she had been advised to follow.

It was hard for me to register the details as she listed them off and even harder to retain them. But they did sound amazingly similar to what I knew of the approach generally recommended for individuals with diabetes. She was quite specific about the various types of sugars and starches she had to regulate.

"And I have to walk every day," she added.

"Is it kind of like those meat-based diets, the high-protein approach?" I asked.

"Oh no, it's not that. Believe me, I've tried that. I've tried every kind of diet there is in my life," she said, and she mentioned several famous ones by name. "Nothing worked. I've tried everything. Everything."

I looked at her in astonishment. This slim woman had tried a million diets in her life? Why?

She read my mind.

"I've lost 120 pounds in the last two years," she said.

"One hundred and twenty pounds!" I couldn't disguise it. I was stunned.

"Oh yes. Ask Marie," she said with a smile, referring to our mutual friend, the mother of the groom. "She knows all about it."

"But I didn't do this to lose weight," she emphasized. "I had to do it, because I was very sick. It's not a weight loss diet. But I did lose weight. Oh, I had tried everything. Ask Marie," she said again, smiling still, as she saw how hard it was for me to imagine her 120 pounds heavier. "Nothing worked for me before."

It was only later that I recalled – and finally understood – her slightly wistful question, later in the evening, when she asked me how was the crème caramel. She had sent it back uneaten, just like the carrot, when the servers cleared the tables at the close of the meal.

As the music started, she entered the dance floor with the happy enthusiasm that seemed to mark her personality in general.

Soon, everyone was dancing. And the great, arching armoury was alive with music and fun as guests of all ages celebrated the enduring importance of a joyful, committed love. Amélie was among the most joyful.

Much later, a long, harvest-style table was spread with yet more desserts. I wandered the length and carefully chose one of the sweet treats to take back to my table to sample. Younger and more energetic dancers sampled as well. Amélie did not.

Watching, participating and celebrating, I mused that the sacrifices, but also the pleasures, of Amélie's new eating habits might well have saved her life; I didn't really know. But if the changes couldn't be framed in quite such extravagant terms, they did seem certainly to have vastly improved its quality. I determined to look up metabolic syndrome and find out just what it was.

Well, I looked it up the next day and on a few other days as well, but I soon determined that metabolic syndrome was well beyond my complete understanding.

The information I found defined it as a cluster of negative health conditions including obesity, high blood pressure, high blood sugar, high bad cholesterol, and low good cholesterol.

I am reluctant to go beyond that in describing it because I cannot offer fulsome information and definitely not advice when it comes to managing this serious medical condition. But there is plenty of information on the internet and in books. I do know that if I had that cluster of symptoms, or was simply heading in that direction, I'd definitely be discussing it with my doctor. And I'd be asking questions about the diet and lifestyle guidelines that worked so well for Amélie.

But this book is not about metabolic syndrome; that is outside my range of expertise.

Suffice to say, however, that nothing about the diet guidelines – as far as I could see – went against the essential diet and lifestyle habits that I have found helpful in my own life. And nothing about them would have surprised my dear, slim, and practical mother in the least!

In fact, she would have been surprised that anyone would actually consider eating in any other way. An approach that values whole foods, sufficient fibre, limits on refined sugar and starch, little if any junk food? What's so special about a diet like that, she would think. This is just normal eating.

Meeting Amélie was an inspiration, offering me an insight into a whole other reason and approach to living slim. Although I never saw her with that additional 120 pounds – or the raised blood pressure, blood sugar and disturbed cholesterol – I do remember Adrianna. I did indeed know her "before" and "after." And she, too, was inspired to finally lose weight because of health considerations – in her case, those of her close family members.

As Amélie said, she had struggled with a multitude of diets for years. Nothing had worked. But now this regime, emphasizing health, not weight loss, had allowed her to become both slim and healthy.

Clearly, it hadn't been all that easy for her to make the change. Clearly, that night in the armoury she would like to have been able to enjoy both that carrot and that crème caramel.

But she had made an important choice. And she'd certainly stuck with it.

And as a sixty-something granny, who could still kick up her heels in a pretty jazzy way on the dance floor, she was looking and feeling great.

CHAPTER 12

Dianne's Story: Cranberries in Alberta

The air in St. Albert, Alberta is to die for.

Fresh and clean, it seems to sweep in from somewhere far away where life is uncomplicated and young.

Or, perhaps I should say uncomplicated and old. Because the northern peaks of the Rocky Mountains with all their grandeur, force, and age are situated several hours further west. And despite the fact that you don't see them as you go about your business in St. Albert, they seem to exist, there in your imagination, permanently, as does the great, massive march of land north of St. Albert, which leads eventually, and seemingly endlessly, towards Canada's north.

My dear friend Dianne lives in St. Albert. And to describe the town more fully, it is a quite typical, somewhat newish, well-ordered, clean, thriving, prosperous, suburban Canadian community just north of Edmonton. It has much in common with countless Canadian communities from one end of this country to the other.

Its origins go back to a small, mainly French, agricultural settlement. But its agricultural beginnings have long since been overwhelmed by the spillover housing needs of the large urban entity that is Edmonton. It is now a thoroughly modern landscape of roads, parks, shopping centres and homes, most of them built on the new and curving suburban streets developed during the last fifty years.

Tall sound barriers block the backyards of some of these homes from the larger arterial roads that intersect the town and that link it seamlessly to Edmonton and the surrounding countryside.

In St. Albert, most people jump in their cars to do *all* their grocery shopping. They jump in their cars to get to work morning, noon, and night. They jump in their cars to go to the doctor, the dentist, and to get their kids to the hockey rink on time. There are no butcher stores at the foot of these winding, subdivision streets. There are no drug stores you can scoot to just around the corner. There are no flower shops a five-minute stroll away.

Long and bitterly cold winters tempt residents to hole up for many months indoors. The West Edmonton Mall, located about 10 minutes away (by car) for most people, pulls everyone (by car) to sample its massive array of shopping, entertainment, over-eating, and recreation options. Massive grocery stores -- super-sized -- offer all the food anyone could possibly desire, all the time.

In other words, and despite its links to a pioneer past, St. Albert is now the essence of modern North American suburbia.

It is exactly what certain urban planners rail against in terms of an environment that encourages healthy active living. It is what some health advocates believe underlies our obesity epidemic. But it is also exactly what many, many Canadians and other

North Americans long for, want, and immensely enjoy as their ideal home base.

How does a Canadian woman stay slim in this environment? Just ask Dianne.

Now in her sixties, with short, wind-blown hair and permanent enthusiasm, Dianne is as slim as she was in her early twenties when she left Edmonton for a few years of work, travel and adventure in big-city Toronto. That is where I met her as she completed her internship as a radiology technician.

Against all life's odds, Dianne carries not one ounce more weight than when she waltzed into work at one of Toronto's busiest hospitals, flashing her infectious smile and sharing her positive attitude, before returning to settle in her home province of big sky, vast spaces, and cheerful ambition.

St. Albert is now where she hangs her hat.

Dianne is of an entirely different generation than my mother. Dianne is of my own generation. Her way of life in suburban St. Albert is a far remove from the life my mother knew growing up, a generation earlier, in St. John's, Newfoundland.

But, in certain fundamental ways, Dianne's daily life choices are closer than you would think to the ones my mother made. They are simple choices and simple decisions that have managed to keep her – like my mother – slim and trim continuously throughout her life.

In my mother's case, we began with the apple. But in this case, we will begin with the cranberry.

Because somehow, somewhere, sometime, Dianne has picked up a fondness for dried cranberries.

Although Christmas dinners for my mother were never complete without her delicious homemade cranberry sauce, the dried (and sugared) cranberries we now enjoy are a relatively recent food product. They were not available in my mother's time.

But almost every salad that graces Dianne's dinner table – and lots of salads grace her dinner table – boasts a sprinkle of dried cranberries. And perhaps a few walnuts. And, if you're lucky, greens that have been pulled from the little vegetable garden she tends in her suburban backyard.

Now the big news here isn't really the fact that Dianne is fond of dried cranberries. And it certainly isn't that some miracle phytonutrient in cranberries will now save your life and ensure you have to think no further about your health. And it isn't even the fact that Dianne gets some of her salad greens from her own backyard.

The news and the point is that Dianne has a habit of valuing, and relishing, and prioritizing the fabulous flavours of fruits and vegetables at her table, echoing my mother's similarly strong habits. And she does it with the choices and flavours and items that she happens to enjoy and that are readily available to her.

Like most Canadian women, Dianne does the great bulk of her food shopping at large grocery chains, not specialty food stores; this is what constitutes mainstream food shopping in our country.

Yes, she does indeed check out a farmers' market that takes place during the summer in St. Albert – one of those places where you feel good as you wander among handcrafted items, picking up fresh corn and heirloom tomatoes. And she may indeed have one favourite place where she likes to buy maple syrup or cheese. But her day-to-day life, her standard, year-round, stock-the-kitchen-shelves efforts are centred around large grocery stores.

I emphasize this because this is the way most of us live in Canada. Most of us base our eating habits around what's offered in our closest chain grocery store.

And, yes, while there are plenty of frozen cheesecakes,

packaged cookies, sugary cereals, and heavily sauced pasta salads in all of these locations, there are also rows and rows of fresh fruits and vegetables, ample supplies of fresh meat, fish and poultry, endless offerings of frozen fish, and shelves of good cereal products. There are also highly nutritious dried fruits and nuts, pulses of wonderful variety and, of course, excellent and reasonably priced dairy products.

These basic ingredients are widely available to most Canadians, with a great deal more variety than was available in my mother's time.

We don't have to have loads of money or shop in specialty shops to eat well and live slim in our country. The trick is in choosing well what goes into our shopping carts.

It certainly helps, as was the case with Adrianna, to know which grocery store departments we might have to avoid: the bread department for some; the aisles with packaged cookies, candy, salted snacks or ice cream for others.

There is no doubt that most Canadians are extremely fortunate to have a great choice and variety of grocery store offerings around which we can build delicious and healthy eating habits.

Dianne's dinner table features all the standard real-food items most Canadians enjoy. But she is exceptionally fond of salads. With cranberries.

Desserts, on the other hand, are rare in Dianne's day-to-day life. Not non-existent. But rare. She turns out a mean apple crumble. But it's a special treat. And let's face it: most Canadian women like to have one or two special desserts up their sleeves to pull out on special occasions.

While desserts don't rank high on Dianne's list of favourite foods, she does have a taste for another form of sugar that was never a part of my mother's life. That would be the sugar contained in glasses of red wine.

One of Dianne's hobbies is wine-making. A cool and quiet space in her basement is dedicated to this interest and many a relaxing and perhaps even contemplative hour is spent there perfecting the results of this interest.

A regular parade of reds – and whites – finds its way from her basement storage racks to join the other items on her dinner table.

This is a fair difference from my mother's meal plans which never needed to consider calories from glasses of wine.

My dear mum grew up far removed from the custom of wine with meals, or, indeed, alcohol of any kind regularly available in the home. On a personal level, I've made a similar choice: not deliberately avoiding the custom but just never finding any form of alcohol all that attractive. As a result, this has been one area of calorie input I've simply never had to think much about.

People who do enjoy their wine and beer may find this as hard to believe as the legions of sweet-eaters who doubt there are those – like one of my daughters – who do not enjoy the taste of sweet.

But this is the case, in my case. The particular tastes and smells of alcoholic beverages do not attract me. They do, however, attract Dianne and they definitely attract many other Canadian women.

Does this difference, in fact, make a difference? Can I still say that Dianne has much in common with my mother's lifelong balancing act in terms of happy, enjoyable slim living?

Well, remember that my mother's approach celebrated the delicious flavours of healthy natural foods, but she also thoroughly enjoyed tea, chocolate, homemade cookies, and desserts. Most of which, like alcohol, are filled with sugar. All of which, like alcohol, offer stimulation to the senses well beyond their nutritional value. But, every one of which she consumed in moderation, ruling her tastes and her appetite carefully and never being over-ruled by them.

Dianne, similarly, clearly relishes the subtleties of flavour and aroma offered by different wines. She loves the ritual, the discipline, and the personal effort she puts into creating her own. I consider it a similar interest to that of my mother and other women of her generation who took pride and pleasure in turning out their perfectly flaky and sweetly delicious blueberry pies.

But what Dianne has, and what my mother had, is that instinctive sense of moderation when it comes to consumption.

Luckily for them, their taste for these stimulants does not run out of control. They enjoy them, savour them even, but they rule these tastes; the tastes never rule them.

Dianne and my mother seem to share this attribute naturally. But it's one I've had to learn and re-learn throughout my life. It's one many of us don't seem to come by completely naturally. But it is learnable. I know that from experience.

What else does Dianne have in common with my mother? An affection for a certain type of regular, inexpensive, all-Canadian outdoor exercise. She walks.

Suburbia may seem set up for cars, not people. But scratch the surface just slightly and you will find many opportunities for walking: trails; parks; sidewalks; and, if all else fails, malls.

Dianne lives very close to a small, green-grassed park. At first glance, it's a rather plain, squared space that seems most suited to kids looking to kick a soccer ball or two. But wait, scratch the surface again; this park has connections. Walk across it and you suddenly link to a pathway that skirts behind backyards, that ends up on a crescent, that loops off a major street, that climbs a bit of a hill, that leads toward another park, that passes by a tiny, perfect lake, that links to another roadway, and that leads neatly and eventually back to Dianne's point of origin.

Dianne knows this drill very well as she takes this walk, or some variation of it, almost every evening with a good friend and the good friend's dog. It takes at least 45 minutes, and they move along at a pretty good clip. Accompanying her takes a bit of effort, as I found out on one recent visit!

But think about it: fresh air, good company, and zero dollars spent on equipment. Could you ask for a better way to exercise? Could you ask, moreover, for a better exercise in mental health?

From the tree-lined streets of Halifax on our Atlantic coast to the flat and spreading beaches of Ontario's Georgian Bay, from the great, green parks of Saskatoon to the endlessly connected ravines of Toronto, Canadian women routinely find beautiful and workable places where they can get out and walk.

With dogs, without dogs. With friends, without friends. Plugged into headsets, or plugged into the natural world around us. On our lunch break, or as part of our commute. We walk.

Yes there's also skiing, swimming, sailing, soccer, skating, curling, mountain hiking, yoga, bowling – and yes, even lawn bowling!! You name it, Canadian women do it. But, as I've said before, and at the risk of being irritatingly repetitious, for many of us who are simply not oriented towards anything more rigorous – or who have only a few minutes during our days to fit something in – walking is the exercise of choice.

Cheap, cheerful, and effective, it was also something that my tiny and mostly sedate mother undertook throughout her life. Not as a power walker to be sure. But simply as a way to move her limbs in the great outdoors, to breathe deeply, to get her blood moving and, frankly, to lift and lighten her mind and mood.

And just because I call it cheap and cheerful doesn't mean

the rich and famous of the world can't see its value. Canada is still a constitutional monarchy, although we rarely stop to think of ourselves that way. Both formally and informally, we maintain many ties to the United Kingdom. None other than the smart and capable woman who heads that country's royal family has been a devoted walker – with her dogs – throughout her life.

Finally, Dianne has another similarity to my mother in that the focus of her life is not now, and never has been, a fixation on remaining slim.

While her trim build is a direct result of certain habits, Dianne's primary focus has always been elsewhere: on cultivating relation-ships (big time); building professional skills; developing personal interests; and offering support to community organizations.

She also instinctively seeks balance, finding her moments of quiet renewal and pause – as my mother did with her famous cups of tea – in her backyard garden, in the quiet activities of her wine-making endeavours, in her friendships and relationships with family, and in her calm ability to set boundaries and replenish her personal strength.

It's not just one thing that has brought Dianne through all these years without one added ounce. And it's certainly not just the cranberries in the salad.

Rather, it's all these habits and approaches working together, played out within the particularities of her life in suburban St. Albert.

While Dianne's tastes, life choices, and approaches to health are unique and individual to her, they're also amazingly similar, in their broad strokes, to those of my mother. A full generation apart, she's still stepping in much the same footsteps, still attuned to much the same truths, and still benefitting from much the same simple but helpful habits.

CHAPTER 13

Lake Memphremagog: Return Again

Lake Memphremagog stretches wide – and sometimes wild when the wind rises – amid the forests, rocky outcrops, towns and occasionally extravagant holiday homes in the region called the Eastern Townships, *les Cantons de l'Est*, just south and east of Montreal.

The nearby ski destination of Mount Orford draws visitors summer and winter while the looming rise of that mountain provides a perfect backdrop to daily life in small-town Magog nestled comfortably on the lake's edge.

For many years now, the area has witnessed a tremendous rise in local agro-businesses. Popular interest in locally produced food – *produits du terroir* – has meant many a *fromagerie* and *vignoble* has been able to thrive, offering exceptional choices in cheese and wine throughout the region.

A steady stream of tourists – Canadian and American – keep

turnstiles clicking and chatter flowing in shops and cafés in Magog and other small towns in the region, especially during the warmer months.

My connection to the area goes back to the teenage years I spent working at a summer camp situated on this lake: two summers in the kitchen prepping food, cooking food, and cleaning pots, pans and tables; one more summer as a camp counsellor, dutifully shepherding my gaggle of kids, some of whom adored the experience, some of whom cried with homesickness, all of whom were sweet and interesting.

It was three summers of experiences I've never forgotten: learning to cook on a near industrial scale; occasionally cooking over open fires on a small, nearby island; horseback riding; swimming; canoeing; sitting around bonfire after bonfire; witnessing the almost drunken explosion of leaping frogs on country roads after a heavy rainfall; and sampling my first bitter taste of black coffee.

All this was interspersed with occasional visits to the nearby town of Magog.

These visits happened when someone had to go to town to purchase supplies. If they coincided with my time-off, I would go along. Once in Magog, I was usually, gloriously, on my own. And I used the time to wander the downtown, get my hair cut, stumble through a bit of French, perhaps purchase some peak-season cherries to eat on a street-side park bench, and also to think. As is the case for most of us, my teenage mind had much to mull over.

A few years ago, I was seized with the sentimental desire to simply lay eyes on the place again. I was in the middle of writing this book and had been struck by the number of times my mind had wandered to this region as I thought about that time in my life: my discovery of English trifle in Sherbrooke; my trip back home through New Brunswick when I'd sampled those crab apple preserves.

Maybe, just maybe, I thought, I would bump into a Dianne, or an Amélie, or another story in the area that I could use in the book.

I was planning a fairly routine trip east to visit family in the Maritimes and decided to go by train rather than air, stopping in Montreal, bussing to Magog, then returning to Montreal again to take the train the rest of the way.

It was spring and when my bus pulled to a stop at the depot just outside Magog, the sight and the smell of those familiar surrounding evergreens prompted immediate memories of camp.

The helpful young taxi driver, who kindly allowed me to use my French, told me about the several places he had worked in different regions of the country before marriage and children made him consider more carefully where he wanted live. Job opportunities might be more limited here, he allowed, but he loved the area and was here to stay.

I knew the region had seen businesses open, close, and open again. Manufacturing is a changing landscape that affects people everywhere. I also knew that some of the town's charming older homes had been turned into *gîtes* – bed and breakfast establishments. In my own charming *gîte*, the talk at the breakfast table was all about new retirement condos nearby.

My first morning there, I set off in random fashion, up this street, down the next, realizing that the pretty and walkable downtown streets were much as I remembered. Suddenly, a different and stronger feeling overcame me: a sense of deeper familiarity. I knew *this* street. I was sure *this* was the spot. And yes, there it was: the same street-side park bench where I'd parked my teenage self almost fifty years ago. And I did indeed sit down again. And I did indeed also think, just like before.

This time though my thoughts were remembering, with a bit of distance, my teenage self, struggling with what I now I understood to be the tiniest bit of excess weight and obsessing far too much over it.

This time, I acknowledged that while I remembered munching on those delicious ripe cherries all those years ago, I also remembered pairing that snack with a personal favourite at the time, digestive biscuits. The digestive label implying they were helpful with digestion; the reality being they were a sweet, starchy, commercial food product very likely made with unhealthy hydrogenated fat. Not the worst of all possible snacks perhaps, but not very healthy either.

How much I had to learn back then. How much I had learned since. I didn't know then that those few extra pounds would shortly turn into quite a few too many. I didn't know then that I would lose those pounds in my mid-twenties through rigorous dieting. I didn't know then that I would slowly gain them again during midlife, and then lose them again, all while discovering and rediscovering the fact that it was the cherries I should keep, and the digestive biscuits I should let go.

I didn't know then that my mother's approach to food – so close to me then that I couldn't see it – would become the path that would eventually allow me to live slim just like her.

I sat on that bench for a while, letting my memories mix and merge with my present day thoughts. It was a good and satisfying moment.

Lunchtime saw me seated in a warm, friendly, little café awash with locals, young people, tourists, the smell of great coffee, and interesting music.

"C'est à ton goût? (It's to your taste?)" asked the server, as

I munched my way through a delicious grilled sandwich of tender chicken, nippy mustard, and savoury vegetables.

"*Oui, bien sûr.* (Yes, absolutely,)" I replied, and we both smiled.

Lingering over coffee, I leafed through magazines, catching up on the life of Céline Dion, thinking what a nice location this would be for a part-time job. No one hurried me to leave.

When I did finally ease out of my comfortable spot, I explored more of the town: stopped into a few shops; toured the lakefront park; popped into the church; and, finally, checked out the large, local, downtown supermarket.

Such supermarket explorations are one of my ongoing habits; I enjoy browsing grocery stores while travelling the way some feel compelled to purchase local newspapers. I remember spending several long minutes staring at adorable little jars of carrot jam and tomato jam in a grocery store in small-town Portugal, knowing I wouldn't find these at home, wondering if I should risk breakage by packing them in my suitcase.

This time in Magog, I looked around, wondering if this was the same place – but evidently and fantastically updated – where I'd made my grocery purchases all those years ago. I honestly couldn't remember. But I think, perhaps, it was.

I checked out the wonderful assortment of cheeses, and purchased a couple of apples chosen from the store's massive and colourful display of produce. I knew I didn't need much to take on my upcoming train trip, but apples, as I may have mentioned, always manage to appeal.

Trips on our cross-country passenger trains in the "sleeper" category come supplied with delightful, fresh meals served at well-set dining tables, morning, noon and night. My husband and I had enjoyed one such trip – a cruise on land, I like to call it – from Toronto to Vancouver and back a few years ago. The memory of those evenings, spent gazing at the vast, encompassing cover of the dark night sky from the comfort of the "panorama" car, will stay with me forever.

That evening, I checked out a local pub just a short walk from my *gîte*.

At the table beside me, a cluster of women friends happily shared food and conversation. At the bar, a constant lively banter unfolded as friend greeted friend and music filled the space. At my table for one, I settled with satisfaction into my thoughts, enjoying that opportunity almost as much as I enjoyed my meal: a perfect and perfectly indulgent serving of crackling fish and chips sided with coleslaw. Let's face it. Some combinations just can't be improved on.

It was a lovely, restful, two-day stay. A sentimental journey, for sure, and one I would think of extending, at some point, into a longer road trip.

But in a twist of timing, it was a memorable part of my present-day life as well.

While there, I received word, via the efficiency of our communication gadgets, that another precious grandchild was on track to enter my life. I'll never forget that moment. That, too, I wouldn't have dreamt of, all those years ago, when my much younger self had no thought of the grandmother I would become.

But all good journeys and all good side trips do come to an end. The bus back to Montreal eventually pulled out with me aboard again.

As we passed those achingly beautiful trees, I reflected that no, I was not able to add a Magogian Dianne or Amélie to this book, despite the many trim women I had noticed going busily about their lives during my stay; despite the healthy eating habits I could assume from some of the shopping decisions I had noticed in the grocery story. I had not wanted to step out of my reflective mood to interview slim women strangers in the pub, along the waterfront, in the café, or at the grocery store. But yes, it was worth it for me to step, for a time, into my own personal past and be there with myself again.

I'm glad I made that sentimental journey. All life is a journey after all. And sometimes it's good to revisit not just our memories but also the places of our youth, and to see them and ourselves as things were then and as things are now.

Several months later in Toronto, in one of those unbelievable, coincidental flukes, a vibrantly energetic and slim acquaintance with no ties whatsoever to Quebec mentioned blithely that she and her husband had decided to retire to a small town in the Eastern Townships, to Magog.

"To Magog," I exclaimed. "Really? To Magog? I know that place."

"Absolutely, to Magog," came the answer.

And the reason?

They had simply taken a driving holiday through the area the previous summer, fallen head over heels in love, and decided that Magog was the place for them.

Sure enough, this past summer the purchase was made. They'll be moving within the year. Bye-bye Toronto. True story.

I told her I'll be coming to visit.

CHAPTER 14

And Finally: Life Itself

The final big and important truth I'd like to acknowledge about healthy weight maintenance for Canadian women is that it should never be the most important thing in our lives.

When our lives become sidetracked or dominated by excess weight, thinking about it, doing something about it, *not* doing something about it, failing at doing something about it can loom large – and sometimes too large – in our thoughts.

I would never say that excess weight should be ignored. It is too significant as a health risk, too much of an irritation and too often a source of depression to just let it go.

However, in thinking about my mother's approach to life, I know that maintaining a slim figure was not so much a goal but rather a by-product of her values, her habits, and her lifestyle.

Like many Canadian women of her time, her love of good food, with all its connections to family and society, enriched her life. But she also knew that life on this amazing earth was larger and more complex than her particular corner of it. My mother knew that making a contribution to society – however large, however small – constituted the essence of personal fulfillment. She may not have used this expression, but the idea that we walk beneath trees that others have planted would have been meaningful to her.

My mother taught school. She felt deeply connected to her family and her friends. She helped many people informally throughout her life. And she loved music.

She was profoundly affected by, and grateful for, the beauty of the natural world. She loved to think about, read about, and discuss societal issues.

These were the parts of her life that meant the most to her, that challenged her, kept her young, and occupied her intellect and her emotions.

Canadian women in every region of our country have a lot going for them in this regard.

We actively participate in the workforce; we read widely; we follow movies, music, television, live performances and the visual arts.

Young and old, we dive with enthusiasm into continuing education.

We hike, we bike, we travel, and we socialize. We socialize *a lot*. We have children. We have pets. We have aging parents. We have nieces and nephews. We volunteer for political parties, environmental groups, neighbourhood improvement efforts, charities, faith groups, block parties, and mum's groups.

And, in our own particular Canadian way, and as do women everywhere, we know how to befriend each other.

Whether we're sixteen or sixty, we understand the importance of one, two, or several "good women friends" in whom we confide, with whom we share our joys and our sorrows, and to whom we turn for support throughout our lives.

This was a tradition, as well, in my mother's time.

Her good school friends remained in touch by letter, across the miles and across the years, throughout her life. One of her sisters became a repeat travel-mate as they took trips together in their later years. A young mother she met in Scotland, during the years she lived there while my dad was furthering his education, remained a close and cherished friend for life.

Friendships like this became even more important as my mother aged.

She helped plan a co-op style dwelling for seniors in Wolfville during her early elder years, and moved there after it was built. It's a lovely place, offering seniors apartments in what looks like a townhouse complex. Beyond it lies the flat and stretching dyke-lands; behind it grows a row of trees including an ancient cherry tree which my mother, ever appreciative of the gifts of nature, tried to harvest, especially when her grandchildren were visiting.

The other residents in this, her later-life home, became both neighbours and good friends. We, her children, were grateful for that.

It was springtime when my mum passed away. She came to her end peacefully and at home. Although she had been experiencing heart issues, her death still came as a shock to her family, her neighbours and her friends. She had been active and independent to the end, continuing her interest in others, in family, and in life itself.

In the days that followed, as my siblings and I made our way through her possessions and our emotions, one of her good friends turned up with a still warm blueberry cake, extending the friendly affection she felt for my mother to us, in a beautiful act of kindness.

This wonderful friendship tradition, often lifelong, continues and is just as strong and perhaps stronger for young Canadian women in our digital age.

Although my own path and the path of many Canadian women toward weight management has been driven by personal efforts, and although it is always personal effort that sustains healthy weight management over the long term, I view some group efforts to be a sort of "friendship" tactic that can be useful for some.

A mother-daughter team I know set out to lose roughly 60 pounds each by joining a well-known group that meets weekly and that routinely promotes a clear and healthy diet plan. The effort paid off very well for the mother, who was well-primed for the effort, but not at all for the daughter.

About a year later, however, that same daughter discovered an app. And that became a different story. The app offered much the same sort of guidance but in a different medium, and also tracked every conceivable health-related aspect of her daily life. It proved to be just the kind of support she needed to eventually mimic her mother's success.

Some may bemoan an apparent physical distancing created by our new methods of communication. I do not.

There are times to set aside our mobile and electronic gadgets, certainly. But as long as they don't trump or replace in-person contact, my observation is that they enhance it. Our species is so incredibly social that it's no wonder our digital social networks have exploded the way they have.

In any event, it is all of these things – not any singular focus on weight – that makes for a fulfilling and rewarding life for Canadian women. I fully salute my mother's approach on this.

Whether we are grabbing a coffee with friends, laying the

groundwork for a farmers' market, writing grant applications for a food bank, getting our kids ready for their first pow wow, researching family history, conjuring the Camino, settling down with a book, tutoring a literacy learner, conducting a choir, or simply calling a loved one on the phone, our interests, our passions, and our commitments need to come first in our lives so that our interest in slimness and health can take its proper place as just one part of a well-lived and satisfying whole.

If I began by talking about "the apple and all of that," and the central role of good food, fresh food, real food, in my mother's home and life, I'll finish by once again giving a nod to that wonderful apple and all the treasures of the earth that it represents.

It is indeed where we must start when we deal with weight management.

But, let's now expand "all of that" to include all of this: those interests, those passions, those friends, those activities that enliven and bring meaning to our lives. Let's go for broke.

Good luck to us all!

ACKNOWLEDGEMENTS

Many thanks to:

My first readers: David Adeney; Brenda Large; Brian Deming; Ian Scott. Their kind words and support meant a lot.

Writing coach Chris Kay Fraser, whose "deep dive" into my stories was intensely helpful.

My cherished family.

ENDNOTES

Page 2
1. https://www.who.int/en/news-room/fact-sheets/detail/
obesity-and-overweight

2. https://www.canada.ca/en/public-health/services/
publications/healthy-living/obesity-excess-weight-rates-
canadian-adults.html

ABOUT THE AUTHOR

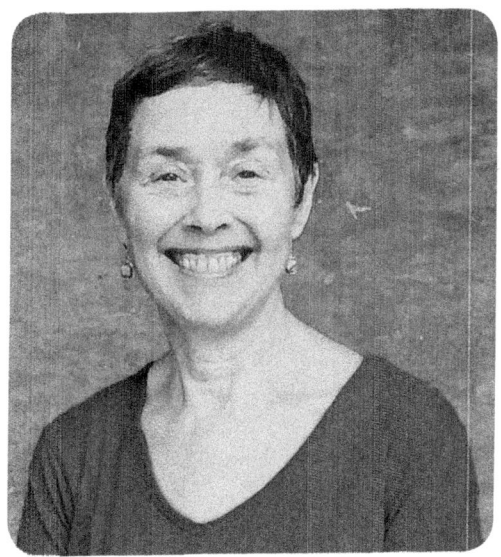

Lillian Salmon grew up on Canada's east coast living in New Brunswick, Nova Scotia, and Newfoundland. Acquiring the slim-living habits of her mother did not come easily to her, but she cherishes the insights gained all the more. She now lives in Toronto with her husband and enjoys spending time with her grandchildren, taking walks in the great outdoors, and sampling wonderful food. This is her first book.

"Today, Nova Scotia's Annapolis Valley remains one of the most delightful places on earth to pick your own blueberries. I am still so in love with these small fruits that, here in Ontario, I buy box after box, all summer long." – **Living Slim: A Canadian Woman's Way**

Purchase **LIving Slim: A Canadian Woman's Way** at:
www.lilliansalmon.com

Printed by BoD™in Norderstedt, Germany